THE
SPICE
LILIES

The
SPICE
LILIES

Eastern Secrets to Healing
with Ginger, Turmeric,
Cardamom, and Galangal

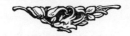

SUSANNE POTH
and
GINA SAUER

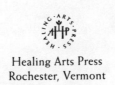

Healing Arts Press
Rochester, Vermont

Healing Arts Press
One Park Street
Rochester, Vermont 05767
www.InnerTraditions.com

Healing Arts Press is a division of Inner Traditions International

*Note to the reader: This book is intended as an informational guide. The
remedies, approaches, and techniques described herein are meant to supple-
ment, and not to be a substitute for, professional medical care or treatment.
They should not be used to treat a serious ailment without prior consultation
with a qualified health care professional.*

LIBRARY OF CONGRESS CATALOGING-IN-PUBLICATION DATA

Poth, Susanne.
    The spice lilies : eastern secrets to healing with ginger, turmeric,
cardamom, and galangal / Susanne Poth and Gina Sauer.
        p. cm.
    ISBN 0-89281-890-5 (alk. paper)
        1. Spices—Therapeutic use. 2. Zingiberaceae. I. Sauer, Gina.
II. Title.

RM666.S64 P68 2000
615'.32—dc21   00-037025

Printed and bound in Canada
10 9 8 7 6 5 4 3 2 1

Text design and layout by Priscilla Baker
This book was typeset in Janson with Weiss as the display typeface

Contents

Preface

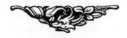

ARE YOU FAMILIAR with ginger and turmeric? Surely you have heard of at least one of these spices in a culinary context. Maybe you have even used them yourself for cooking or baking. But did you know that you were dealing with actual medicines as well? In this book we want to present the medical as well as the culinary aspects of the ginger family. That is why we wrote the book together. One author is a pharmacist and an expert on healing plants. She will inform you about the positive effects of turmeric and ginger on the digestive system, the circulatory system, the immune system, the joints, and much more. The other author is a sociologist, passionate about cooking with ginger. She will inform you about the cultural history of the spice lilies. All of the recipes in this book come from her personal repertoire; she invented several of them herself.

Even though both of us are fans of the spice lilies, we recognize that spice preference is ultimately a matter of taste. Not everyone will share our enthusiasm. Those who do not like ginger and turmeric should not force themselves to eat them just because they are healthy. After all, it can't be healthy to eat something you don't like. Furthermore, there are almost always alternatives. But to those who avoid the spice lilies out of concern that they might not digest them well, we can offer some reassurance: not only are ginger, turmeric, galangal, and cardamom easily digestible, but they improve the digestion of other foods. That is why they occupy a prominent place in healthy cooking.

To the healthy and the sick, the gourmets and those that want to become gourmets, we wish an enjoyable time reading this book.

Susanne Poth and Gina Sauer

I

The Ancient Global Spice Trade

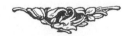

ALL THE HIGHLY DEVELOPED ancient cultures in Egypt, China, India, and Mesopotamia used spices. Cooks refined their meals with them, priests burned them to honor the gods with their scent, and doctors prescribed them as medicine. But not all spices could be cultivated in every locale. For centuries, ginger and turmeric grew only in Southeast Asia.

The home of wild ginger and turmeric is Malaysia. Cardamom is native to Sri Lanka and southern India. The small galangal comes from China, the big galangal from Sumatra. Southeast Asian traders brought these spices to northern India and even to East Africa as early as the second millennium B.C.E. The Indians were eager dealers and seafarers as well. They took spices from the Indus valley to Arabia and Mesopotamia. Over the centuries these sought-after goods even made it to Europe. The Romans and Greeks were as familiar with these spices as were their ancestors in Egypt, Akkad, and Sumer.

The Ginger Family in Mesopotamia

Cardamom was well liked in ancient Babylon. The warrior-king Merodachbaladan pursued a peaceful hobby in his spare time; he was a horticulturist. In the eighth century B.C.E. he wrote the world's first book on horticulture, with long lists of plants and botanical descriptions. The king had sixty-four types of plants in his garden, including saffron, thyme, coriander, and cardamom.

Ginger and turmeric were used in Mesopotamia as well but were not cultivated there. The Assyrian king Ashurbanipal commissioned a report on these plants around 650 B.C.E. The report appears in what may have been the largest library of ancient times. On about 30,000 clay tablets the king preserved and passed down the knowledge of his times. The tablets list about 250 healing plants and spices. Ginger and turmeric are listed especially as brewing spices and as stomach tonics. They also appear with saffron and sumac in the category of dye plants.

The Assyrians used Turmeric to obtain the color yellow, saffron for orange, and sumac for purple. To this day fresh turmeric is applied to palms in the Near East. While this practice has no specific medical value, it is said to contribute to overall well-being.

Those that have had a turmeric bulb in their house know that the slightest contact with the intensely orange, juicy root leads to bright yellow stains on hands, towels, and counters. The color is not water soluble but is easily removed with an oil-soaked towel or alcohol. Moreover, the stains fade out over time with exposure to light.

Ginger, on the other hand, has no coloring characteristics. Nonetheless, on the Assyrian tablets ginger and turmeric both appear in the category of dye plants. Thus the Assyrians clearly believed that the two bulbs belonged to the same botanical family. Ginger does not have its own name in Syrian but is instead called *kurkanu sa sadi*, which means "turmeric from the mountains." Which mountains do they mean?

The ancient Syrians were not very familiar with the home of the two spices. Huge land masses separated their country from the Indus valley. Those that made the overland trek to India had to cross many mountains. Beyond these mountains lay the land in which the two spices originated. Trade relations between Mesopotamia and India can be traced all the way back to 3000 B.C.E.

The Ginger Family in China

Ginger, galangal, cardamom, and turmeric played an important role in ancient China. They were important not only as scents for the gods and spices for cooking, but also as medicine. The first teaching of Chinese herbal medicine is attributed to Schen Nong, one of the three most famous Chinese emperors, who included plants from the ginger family in his pharmacopoeia. He is believed to have lived around 2700 B.C.E. The oldest version of his teachings was recorded around the time of the birth of Christ by an unknown group of Chinese doctors, thus documenting a period of roughly 2700 years. During this time Shen Nong's teaching was further developed and passed on by many wise herbalists.

Schen Nong is considered the "celestial horticulturist." He divided plants into three groups: Those called "helper drugs" were prescribed carefully and only in case of acute illness. Plants that belonged to the middle group were called "minister drugs," they could have some negative side effects and were generally prescribed to ameliorate nutritional deficiencies. The highest medicines were called "ruler drugs." Regardless of their dosage they would never be toxic and were prescribed to nurture life. Ginger and galangal belonged to this group and both were considered to exhibit warming characteristics.

The Ginger Family in India

The Indians have also known the members of the ginger family for millennia. It is impossible to imagine Indian cuisine without ginger, cardamom, and turmeric, while galangal is of greater culinary significance in Southeast Asia and China.

Turmeric has always had a double function. It spiced dishes while at the same time coloring them. Curry powder, hot spicy dishes, mustard, and pickled vegetables are all colored yellow-orange by turmeric. Even the robes of monks were colored with turmeric, since yellow-orange is also the symbolic color of Hinduism. Turmeric is a well-known and affordable plant dye that to this day occupies a prominent place in India's culture and everyday life.

The medicinal usage of ginger and turmeric is recorded in the *Sushruta Samhita*, a historic collection of medical texts spanning at least nine centuries. It is the basis of modern ayurvedic medicine. Ayurveda, along with traditional Chinese medicine, belongs to the oldest healing systems in the world and is still practiced today. The oldest remaining edition of the *Sushruta Samhita* was written down in about the second century C.E. Its sources, however, stretch back to the seventh century B.C.E. During this time ayurvedic healing was further developed by many authors.

Ginger was and is one of the main components of ayurvedic medications. Trikatu, "the three spicy ones," is the name of a classic mixture of ginger, black pepper, and longpepper (*Piper longum*, also known as pippali). While turmeric does belong to the family of spice lilies, it is classified as a bittering substance and not, like ginger, as a spicy medication.

How the Spice Lilies Got Their Names

Ginger, galangal, turmeric, and cardamom are also referred to as spice lilies. Their names come from the Sanskrit vocabulary of ancient India.

GINGER

Ginger in Sanskrit is *sringavera*, "antler-shaped." According to more recent research, *sringavera* is supposed to have referred only to the dried root, the commonly traded form. The word is well chosen, dried ginger resembles antlers much more than it does when fresh.

GALANGAL

At first only the big galangal from Indonesia was known in India. The small galangal from China came later. In order to differentiate between the small and the big galangal , the Chinese called the big galangal *kao liang kiang*. *Kao* means "big." The Indians kept the prefix and invented the Sanskrit word *kulanja*, and the Greeks transformed it into *galanga*.

TURMERIC
(Curcuma)

The word for turmeric also derives from the Sanskrit. There it was called *cuncuma*, in Assyrian *kurkanu*, and in Arabic *kurkum*. It finally became the Latin word *curcuma*. The etymology of the word, however, posed a mystery for linguists for a long time, as the expensive and much desired saffron was also once called *cuncuma*. Saffron, which consists of deep orange aromatic stigmas from a purple crocus, was and remains today an expensive spice. It probably originated in Greece or the Middle East and was traded from the West to the East. It is considered as desirable and valuable in Asia as in Arabia or Europe.

Originally the word *cuncuma* designated only the coloring characteristics of the plants. But this created confusion and led to fraud. Cheap ground turmeric was called *cuncuma*, as was expensive ground saffron. That is why turmeric has sometimes been called "fake" or "Indian" saffron, even though these spices have, apart from their color, little in common.

Sometimes in Indian cookbooks, saffron is written when turmeric is meant. Aside from that, one should not substitute turmeric for saffron when cooking. A bouillabaisse, a Milanese risotto, or a paella, for which "real" saffron is indispensable, can be converted into a horrible curry dish with turmeric, as the other ingredients are not compatible.

The Home of the Spice Lilies

The ancient Indians named the individual members of the spice family. Their language, Sanskrit, is the mother of almost all European languages, so that the origin of their names can be recognized to this day. India, however, is not the home of these wild plants.

Seafarers from Southeast Asia brought ginger, cardamom, and turmeric to India, and even to the coast of North Africa, long before people in these areas succeeded in cultivating these plants.

Southeast Asian sailors traveled west across the Indian ocean in the second millennium B.C.E. and "discovered Africa." Long before the Arabs and the Europeans ventured onto the high seas, they used the monsoon winds and sailed in simple boats out into the open ocean. They did not need a compass for navigation, as they knew how to interpret the temperature of the water, the patterns of the waves, the stars, the sun, and when the skies were cloudy the directionally constant deep sea lightning (the origins of which remain a mystery to this day) led the way.

This route to East Africa quickly expanded into a trade route—the so-called cinnamon route, since cinnamon was the Southeast Asians' most important trading product. They landed on Madagascar and Zanzibar and traded the cinnamon for glass, bronze, clothing, and jewelry. The fleet of the Pharaohs sailed toward them for a stretch of the East African coast. Egyptian priests needed cinnamon for their ceremonies and the embalming of their dead. Along with the cinnamon, ginger came to East Africa, although the sailors initially carried the plant for very different reasons. Sailors on these trips brought ginger along mainly for their own consumption, just like their colleagues from India and China. They knew from experience that it was a good thing to have on board—those who ate it did not get seasick even in the worst of weather.

The Spice Lilies in Classical Greece and Rome

Many famous classical authors wrote about the members of the spice lily family. But at first they wondered what ginger, galangal, turmeric, and cardamom actually looked like. Surely one knew what the dried plant looked like, but for some time the appearance of the fresh plant was not known in the West. That is why the plants that Alexander the Great brought back from his expedition to India created a veritable sensation.

Theophrastus, a great botanist and contemporary of Alexander the Great, classified all plants known in his time, including the souvenirs from India. He recognized the warming quality common to ginger, cardamom, and turmeric and was the first Greek to group them together in a plant family.

Classical physicians used the spice lilies most commonly to treat poisoning and stomach troubles. Greek and Roman cuisine also featured the spice lilies for their good flavor. Thus they became a component of many recipes.

THREE JOURNEYS TO SOMALIA

Marcus Gavius Apicius, a famous Roman epicure, spiced gravies and marinades with cardamom seeds and ginger powder. This must have been very healthy for him as he lived to the age of ninety-five, dying in 37 C.E. Galangal, on the other hand, is missing from his recipes as it was still unknown in Europe in his time. He was also unaware of fresh ginger but once came very close to it. He traveled to Somalia once because there were supposed to be large crabs on the coast there. The voyage was a disappointment. The African crabs were no larger than the Italian ones, so Apicius traveled back to Rome without leaving the ship. He thus missed the opportunity to buy a few pieces of fresh ginger from the natives.

Pliny the Elder, a Roman natural scientist, was familiar with ginger. When he visited Roman ports in Somalia he saw ginger in cultivation there. In his famous *Historia naturalis* he reports that ginger, in spite of its spicy flavor, goes bad quickly. He also dispelled the notion, held until then, that ginger was the root of the pepper tree. Pliny also described cardamom. He divided cardamom seeds into four categories based on quality. The best quality seed was green, was difficult to break, and had hard sharp edges.

Dioscorides, Nero's personal doctor, recommends the same characteristics for selecting cardamom. "Choose that which is hard to be broken" is what he wrote in his famous book *De materia medica*, which contains the botanical and pharmaceutical knowledge of his times. Dioscorides also had experience with fresh ginger. He loved the fine scent of the plant and, like Theophrastus, attributed warming qualities to it. He too traveled to Somalia and saw how natives on the coast grew ginger for their personal use. They added the young sprouts raw to salads or chewed them by themselves. They used the more mature sprouts for boiling water for distillation and also in the preparation of warm food. They dried the oldest parts of the root and shipped them to Italy.

Hard Times for the Spice Lilies

After the division of the Roman empire in 476 C.E. all the desirable spices of the East were available in Byzantium. Only galangal was still unavailable in European markets. Only in the sixth century C.E. did the doctor Aëtius of Amida write about the root, the first and only author of antiquity to do so.

Following the fall of Rome, trade stagnated in the West. The countries of the barbarians fell into the state that earned the early Middle Ages the adjective "dark." Only the Christian monks continued to cultivate and study healing plants and spices. It wasn't until the tenth century C.E. that Arab and Jewish traders began to bring more spices to Europe.

The doctor Ibn Jaqub visited the German city Mainz in 973 C.E. and was pleased that here "the spices of the Far East are common, while the city lies in the dark West." He looked through the shelves of Mainz merchants and found pepper, ginger, and galangal in their inventory.

The abbot and healing expert Hildegard von Bingen knew galangal and ginger. Whether to stimulate the appetite, to treat eye ailments, or relieve stomach colics, she could rely on the spice lilies. But she also feared their heat. She discouraged healthy, well-fed people from their consumption. She considered ginger in particular to make people lazy, clumsy, and forgetful. She believed that ginger increased animalistic tendencies in people and destroyed reason. Thus Hildegard von Bingen was among the few that warned against the consumption of ginger.

Cooking in the Middle Ages— The Comeback of the Spice Lilies

If you look at spice consumption in the late European Middle Ages, you will realize that spices were used about a hundred times more than they are today. Does that mean that the cooks back then constantly overspiced their dishes?

An exceptionally detailed recipe with all quantities spelled out comes from Monsieur Chiquart, a French chef of the fifteenth century. He calls for about three hundred pounds of ginger, pepper, cinnamon, and cardamom. But these are only the main spices. Saffron, muscat, cloves, dates, stone-pine seeds, almonds, plums, raisins, sugar, and figs amounted to another several pounds.

At first glance, many recipes did indeed call for unbelievable amounts of spices. But to calculate their relation to the food being seasoned, one needs to know the exact quantities of all the ingredients. These, however, are missing from most recipes. One thing is certain; the original recipes from the Middle Ages were not designed for a family dinner but, rather, for a royal feast. Such a feast would last several days. Several hundred animals would be slaughtered, and huge amounts of vegetables would be offered as side dishes. So it stands to reason that large quantities of spices would be required to make all this palatable.

In Monsieur Chiquart's recipe all these ingredients were used to tenderize and spice about seventy thousand pounds of meat. When all quantities of the recipe are compared, the ratio turns out to be one part spices to one hundred parts other ingredients. That's about the same proportions as in a well-spiced Asian dish nowadays.

Goodbye, Spice Lilies

In the seventeenth century spices lost their attraction. Cooks discovered the taste of the actual ingredients and only used spices sparingly. The French, especially, banned spices from their recipes. As French cuisine became the international role model, spices lost their good reputation all across Europe. Ginger and cardamom were barely able to secure themselves a small role as a cookie spice. In the eighteenth and nineteenth centuries tea, coffee, cocoa, and sugar were the engines behind world trade.

How the Spice Lilies Came to America

As early as the sixteenth century Spanish and Portuguese sailors began bringing spices from Indonesia to the Caribbean, to cultivate them there and export them to Europe later. Reportedly, the plantation owners in the Caribbean exported about one million tons of ginger to Europe in 1547. When the Spanish and Portuguese left, the Far Eastern spice plantations stayed behind. Thus Caribbean cuisine melded with Asian cuisine. Both Asian and Caribbean cuisines have influenced North American cuisine for some time now. Having realized how healthy they are, many modern American people have adapted their diets to include the spice lilies. A healthier lifestyle includes more vegetables, more exercise, and fewer calories— with spices lean meats and vegetables taste good too. An adventurous spirit helps, which further explains the comeback of the ginger family. Numerous Chinese, Indian, Vietnamese, Caribbean, and Thai restaurants flourish in North America, and ever increasing rates of travel support the trend to the exotic. Since the early 1990s ginger, galangal, turmeric, and cardamom have been available in Asian grocery stores in all major American cities. The products are fresh, cheap, and of good quality. All friends of the ginger family can only hope that it will stay this way forever.

JAKE LEG BLUES

A sad episode in the history of ginger occurred in the United States in 1930. Some American newspapers brought reports of a new ailment; thousands of Americans suddenly found their legs becoming paralyzed. Recovery was very slow, and in some cases the nervous system did not recover at all. At first doctors believed they were dealing with polio, an infectious disease caused by a virus. But after closer examination they realized that the symptoms were different.

A short time later the true culprit was found. It was a liquid extract of Jamaican ginger, known as "Jake," that was sold in pharmacies as a digestive aid and headache remedy. As prohibition was in effect at the time, drinking alcohol was illegal. But Jake, although it contained 70 percent alcohol, was classified as a medication and was therefore a legal substance. As such, it became highly sought after for recreational purposes.

The medicine was not considered palatable because of its strong ginger taste, but necessity is the mother of invention. Desperate people tried to cover the taste with Coca Cola or lemonade. The high-proof ginger medicine sold quickly and became a hit. Small wonder then, that fake ginger medicines began to appear on the market, produced with sugar syrup, castor oil, or glycerin to counteract the taste. But these substances were not the cause of the paralysis. Doctors finally figured out that the disease was caused by the 2 percent addition of a chemical solution called triortho-cresylphosphate. The substance was cheap and dissolved readily into the alcohol and ginger extract solution. But at the time, the manufacturers didn't realize that the combination was toxic.

The victims formed a consumer group in the hopes of receiving financial compensation from the government, but to no avail. The incident, which was recorded in medical history under the name Jamaican Ginger Paralysis, is also remembered in many pop songs with titles such as "Jake Leg Blues" or "Jake Walk Papa."

A Botanical Family Portrait

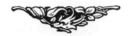

GINGER, TURMERIC, cardamom, and galangal all belong to the ginger plant family, or *Zingiberaceae*. The members of the ginger family are closely related to the lily plants botanically and, for this reason, are sometimes referred to as "spice lilies." All four plants belong in the kitchen of any real spice fan. But they can also be found in any well-stocked homeopathic pharmacy. What do these plants have in common, and what sets them apart from one another? A short excursion into the world of botany helps answer these questions.

GINGER

The knotty yellow growth that we buy as fresh ginger root is only the subterranean part of a reedlike stem that lives for one year. Each year a new stem grows from the rootstock, reaching from three to six feet in height. The stem consists of leaf bases that are stacked closely together. Each leaf is about seven inches long, is narrow, and has a tip that resembles a lance. Very rarely a second stem will extend to the side, topped with a decorative blossom that consists of many small petals resembling orchids. Once pollinated (the pollen is usually spread by birds), the blossom will develop into a capsule with several seeds. But the ginger plant flowers only rarely, and propagation by seeds is not necessary for its cultivation. Instead, ginger is propagated by root division. This means that a suitable piece of the root will simply be divided and stuck into the earth. Each piece will give rise to a new and complete ginger plant. This process is referred to as vegetative (asexual) reproduction.

The meaty, yellow ginger bulb is called a rhizome. This subterranean rootstock is the plant's storage organ for the winter. The rhizome is about three to seven inches long and one inch wide, dented on the sides, and branched off like antlers. It is divided into several fanlike parts. With its short, thick fingers it is sometimes referred to as a ginger "hand." It is surrounded by a thin bark, with flaky leaf scars circling the structure. Thin roots extend downward but these are removed after harvest.

The ginger rootstock produces new green sprouts under earth continually, from which one-year stems grow. The older parts of the rhizome eventually die off, thus over time the plant crawls closely along the surface.

ROOT AND ROOTSTOCK

Because they both grow under the earth and look fairly similar, root and rootstock are often confused. However, they have very different functions. While both can store nutrients, only the root can take in nutrients such as nitrogen, sulfur, and phosphorus from the ground. The rootstock's function is similar to the stem's function above earth—it generates the leaves. That is why it is sometimes also referred to as the "earth sprout." The relationship between sprout and earth sprout becomes very apparent under the microscope as the structure of the two is very similar. But even with the naked eye several similarities can be observed: on the rhizome one sees regressed leaves surrounding the rootstock like flakes, a characteristic that is not shared by the root.

TURMERIC
(Indian Saffron, Long-Rooted Curcuma)

Turmeric is also known as "curcuma." Botanically, it is called *Curcuma domestica*, and it originates in Southeast Asia. Turmeric is a low-growing plant with petiolate leaves that are between three and seven feet long. In aspect it is reminiscent of a banana plant. As with ginger, a separate stem bears the dense, yellow petals. Again as with ginger, the rootstock is the most interesting part of the plant for culinary and medical purposes. It is knotty and thick with numerous fingerlike side rhizomes. After the leaves wilt, the yellow to reddish brown rhizome and the side bulbs are dug out, cooked briefly, peeled, and dried.

Aside from *Curcuma domestica*, *Curcuma zanthorrhiza*, also known as Java turmeric, is also of pharmaceutical significance. It is cultivated mainly in Java and other parts of Indonesia. Botanically speaking, it is almost identical to its Indian counterparts.

GALANGAL

This plant, which reaches a height of up to six feet, is also a typical representative of the ginger family. Its official names are *Alpina officinarum* for the small variety and *Alpina galanga* for the big galangal. Galangal comes from southern China, India, and Thailand. Its leaves are one foot long and one inch wide and have lancelike tips. The white petals are attached at the end of the stem like grapes. As with ginger and turmeric, only the rootstock is useful for culinary and medicinal purposes. It is considerably smaller than the rootstock of ginger.

CARDAMOM
(Green Cardamom)

The plant with the Latin name *Elettaria cardamomum* comes from the southwestern Malabar Coast of India. It is cultivated there as well as in southern India, Sri Lanka, Java, and Guatemala. The plant grows from seven to thirteen feet tall and has leaves about two feet long that narrow down to lancelike tips. In this ginger family plant, the useful spice is for once not found in the rootstock but, rather, in the seeds. The plant produces one-inch-long capsule fruits that are harvested shortly before they ripen. In order to keep the seeds from losing their aroma during drying and storage, they are left in their natural protective coating, the capsule, until ready for use. This natural packaging also keeps Malabar cardamom from being mixed with other lower grade types of cardamom, for example the long or Ceylon cardamom *(Elettaria major)*, or the Bengal cardamom *(Amomum aromaticum)*. "Grains of paradise" *(Aframomum melegueta)* are the seeds of another ginger family plant. They look very similar to cardamom seeds but have a reddish brown color. Although this spice was once, as the name suggests, very valuable, it is no longer significant in the Western world today and is very hard to obtain.

The Right Chemistry

In large part, the fresh rhizomes of ginger, galangal, turmeric, and fresh cardamom seeds are composed of water, starch, protein, raw fibers, and fats. In addition, they contain small amounts of vitamins, which are nutritionally speaking insignificant as the plants are ingested in relatively small amounts, either as spices or as medicine. Minerals do not appear in significant quantities either. What is noticeable, though, is the low sodium content of these spices.

NUTRITIONAL COMPOSITION OF THE DRIED SPICES

Nutritional Constituents	Ginger	Turmeric	Cardamom	Galangal
Water %	10.0	9.5	8.0	10.0
Protein %	9.0	8.0	11.0	9.0
Fat %	6.0	10.0	6.5	6.5
Carbohydrate %	71.0	64.0	69.0	70.0
Raw fiber %	6.0	6.5	11.0	7.0

ACTIVE INGREDIENTS OF THE PLANTS

Volatile Oils %	1.0–3.0	2.0–5.0	3.5–8.0	0.5–1.5
Other Ingredients	Spicy constituents: gingerol, shogaol	Yellow coloring: curcumin and bittering substances	–	Strong-tasting resins: alpinol, galangol, and tannins

The constituents that give these plants their characteristic spiciness and medical strength make up only a fraction of their weight. These so-called secondary plant ingredients give the plants their botanical and culinary value. From a botanical standpoint, plants produce these secondary ingredients as defenses, to keep from being eaten by grazing animals, or to keep other plants from growing too closely. The members of the ginger family are known for containing larger amounts of volatile oils than plants in most other families. In addition, some members of the family also have strong-tasting ingredients, bittering substances, and tannins. These are the following:

GINGER ROOTSTOCK

If ginger is extracted with solvents such as alcohol, and if the extracting liquid is then carefully steamed away, a golden balsamic resin remains behind. This resin, called oleoresin, makes up between 5 and 8 percent of the rhizome. Oleoresin is one third liquid volatile oils, and another third spicy constituents. The remaining constituents are fats and other organic substances.

The volatile oils are deposited mainly under the bark of the bulb. They are a mixture of monoterpines (for example, limonene, myrcene, phellandrene, pinene, neral, citral) and sesquiterpines (for example, zingiberene, bisabolene, curcumin). Together, they give ginger its characteristic aroma.

The mild, almost sweet flavor comes from the spicy constituents. In ginger it is mostly gingerol and shogaol. The latter was named "shoga" by the Japanese researcher who discovered the constituent, "shoga" being the Japanese name for ginger. The shogaol, which is considerably spicier than the gingerol is hardly present in the freshly harvested root. It is produced only during drying and storage and becomes more pronounced with cooking through the extraction of water. That is why ginger, as opposed to most spices, does not lose flavor from cooking but, rather, becomes more spicy. However, this magic has its limits: storing the ginger for too long or under improper conditions, or cooking it improperly, causes the spicy shogaol to break down into organic combinations that lose the characteristic spiciness entirely. Volatile oils, which are responsible for ginger's aroma, also suffer from lengthy cooking or storage.

WHAT ARE SPICY CONSTITUENTS?

On our tongues there are specific taste buds for every taste. We taste bitter at the base of the tongue, sour on the sides, salty a little further to the front, and sweet on the tip of the tongue. However, there are no taste buds for spiciness. Nevertheless, we still sense spices clearly because the spicy constituents stimulate the warmth and pain receptors of the mucous membranes, thus stimulating digestion and many other bodily processes.

GALANGAL ROOTSTOCK

In spite of the close relationship between galangal and ginger, galangal receives far less attention in Western cuisine and medicine than ginger does. Galangal is considered a "mild brother," but it does have its own unique character. The Sanskrit word for the plant, *sugandha*, means "good-smelling." The galangal rhizome has a sweet, spicy smell. The fresh rhizome smells a bit like pine needles, the dried more like cinnamon. Galangal too contains most volatile oils from the sesquiterpine group, as well as pinene, eugenol, camphor, cinnamaldehyde, and a strong-tasting resin. It also contains a group of spicy constituents, which for simplicity's sake are here combined under the term "galangol," as was commonly done in the past. Furthermore, there is gingerol in the rhizome as well. Other ingredients are tannins and up to 25 percent starch.

CARDAMOM SEEDS

It is quite surprising that a spice with such an intense taste and such a fine aroma receives so little attention in Europe and North America today. Malabar cardamom has a sweet, spicy, slightly biting taste, which gives gingerbread and spiced cookies their characteristic flavor.

A content of up to 9 percent volatile oils in the seed is the source of cardamom's flavor. These are mainly cineole, terpinyl acetate, limonene, sabinenes, and borneol. Even though these components can be found in many plants, they are present in cardamom in such a specific combination that the seeds have an irreplaceable taste. Aside from the volatile oils the seed also contains large amounts of starch and lipids.

TURMERIC ROOTSTOCK

The turmeric rhizome smells good and has a strong taste of resin that is slightly spicy when fresh. When the rootstock is dried, it develops a spicy aroma, which becomes stale after prolonged storage. The various turmeric types are rich in volatile oils and curcumin. The highest content is found among plants that are about six months old. At six months the plant has almost reached its full height and the leaves are still fresh and green. But the rootstock hasn't stored a lot of starch yet, so the plant shrinks substantially during drying. That is why plants are not harvested until later when their cells are filled with starch. In Nepal, the curcumin content of the plant is determined on a weekly basis from the time that the leaves begin to wilt, until they die off completely. They harvest the rhizomes when the optimal relation between the various components is reached. This relation lies at about 30 to 40 percent starch (in regard to the weight of the dried rootstock), 3 to 5 percent volatile oils, and 4 to 6 percent curcumin.

Sesquiterpines such as alantolactone, curlon, and tumeron (which is responsible for the characteristic scent) are the main ingredients of the volatile oils. Further ingredients are zingiberenes, curcumol, and small amounts of cineole, sabinenes, and borneol. Researchers sometimes speak of curcuminoids, curcuminlike substances. Their structure resembles that of spicy constituents but they do not have a spicy taste. For example, the most characteristic ingredient of the bright yellow turmeric root is curcumin, which, however, is only one component of a mixture of chemically similar substances. Rather than tasting spicy, turmeric has a slightly bitter taste. A typical characteristic of the curcumin complex is the yellow to reddish color, which makes it a less costly alternative to saffron.

3

Ginger, Turmeric, Cardamom, and Galangal— Spices As Medicine

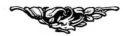

IT IS DISTURBING to see how many households even today use salt as the only seasoning. Aside from the fact that this practice gives the food a monotonous flavor, salt is known to be more harmful than helpful for our health. There are thousands of fabulous spices that not only enhance the flavor of food but enhance our health as well. However, many consumers remain unaware of them. This chapter is intended to show how the plants of the ginger family have great potential to keep you healthy, and even to alleviate minor ailments.

In Asian healing practices, as well as in ayurvedic medicine, ginger, turmeric, cardamom, and galangal have been important ingredients for millennia. American and European scientists have become curious about these plants as well. They are trying to find scientific ways to explain the effectiveness of these plants. They have been aware for some time that these plants are more than merely exotic flavorings.

Medicine for the Stomach and the Intestines

Digestion is not exclusively a matter of the stomach and intestines. A good digestion begins with seeing and smelling a meal. These perceptions determine whether saliva will be secreted in the mouth. The digestive process begins with chewing the food and mixing it with saliva in the mouth. The final goal of digestion is to break the meal down into its nutritional components, carbohydrate, protein, and fat, to be distributed by the blood throughout the body. Food that is not properly broken down in the mouth stays in the stomach and intestines for a long time.

The partially broken-down food travels from the mouth to the stomach through the esophagus. In the stomach it is mixed thoroughly with stomach acid. Stomach acid contains salt, acid, and enzymes, a special mixture that breaks the food down further. While the food mixes with the digestive juices, muscles transport it to the pylorus, the exit of the stomach, and slowly pass it on to the intestines.

This marks its start through a tunnel that is six meters long from beginning to end, the inner surface of which would cover the area of a tennis court—about two hundred square meters—if it were flattened out. The entire inner mucuous membrane of the small intestine is lined with intestinal villi, a multitude of minute finger-shaped processes. In this way the digestive organ offers more area of contact for nutrient absorption into the bloodstream than a smooth surface would provide. In the first part of the intestine, the duodenum, the food is enriched with digestive juices from the gallbladder and the pancreas and is further decomposed. In the longest tract, the small intestine, the food, which by now is broken down into its various nutritional components, is absorbed into the bloodstream and passed throughout the body by the circulatory and lymph systems. The food is absorbed as fats, proteins, carbohydrates, vitamins, minerals, and water.

In the next section, the large intestine, bacteria work on the solid food that has yet to be broken down, decomposing the undigested food particles with fermentation and excretory processes. A healthy balance of beneficial intestinal bacteria is not only important for good digestion but also protects against harmful bacteria. In the large intestine more water is extracted from the remaining solids, leaving a thicker mass. In this way the body regains a large part of the fluid it had added to the food in the form of digestive juices. In the final part of the large intestine, the rectum, the remaining contents collect—held back by a constricting muscle, the anal sphincter—to be excreted on demand.

General tips for good digestion: Take your time when cooking, and especially when eating. Try not to be distracted from the business at hand. TV and heated discussions should not be part of dinner, as they interfere with digestion. Avoid eating too much fat, do not eat too late in the evening, and help your stomach with digestion by adding beneficial spices.

SPICE LILIES HELP DIGESTION

The strength of ginger, turmeric, cardamom, and galangal lies in the digestive process. Thus it is no surprise that they have been used since ancient times as digestive aids. In ginger it is especially the spicy constituents that improve digestion: the gingerol and the shogaol, which only form during cooking or drying. They activate warmth receptors in the mucous membrane of the mouth and in the stomach encouraging the production of saliva and stomach juices. These fluids contain enzymes that break down the food and make its nutrients accessible. Ginger stimulates circulation in the stomach as well, which also enhances digestion.

The spicy constituents of the ginger as well as the active ingredients of turmeric also stimulate the production of bile and thereby facilitate digestion. Bile is formed in the liver and injected directly into the duodenum. Bile breaks down fats into smaller fat particles that can be absorbed by the mucous membrane of the small intestine. The remainder of the bile is collected in the gallbladder and thickened. If the liver does not produce enough bile, fat digestion will be difficult.

The sixteenth-century physician Paracelsus described the effectiveness of turmeric in the treatment of gallbladder ailments. From turmeric's yellow color he deduced that it would be effective for gallbladder ailments, as the color of bile is yellow also. It is probably just a coincidence that in this case the "signature teaching" of Paracelsus was in accord with reality. However, his findings are confirmed by modern medicine: both types of curcumin, turmeric and Java turmeric, increase the excretion of bile (choleretic) and also stimulate the emptying of the gallbladder (cholekinetic). Researchers ascribe these effects mostly to the sesquiterpine curcumin and to curcuminlike complexes.

Bile is a laxative as well, so it is easy to explain why turmeric helps solve other digestive problems. Especially among elderly people, liver and gallbladder functioning is reduced. This is one possible explanation as to why elderly people are more prone to constipation and related ailments. Unfortunately, they are often reluctant to try exotic spices because they think that they will be hard to digest. In fact, it would be very beneficial for them to use more of the healthy spices from the spice lily family in their meals to stimulate digestion.

The important medical significance of turmeric is shown in epidemiological studies, according to which gallbladder ailments on Java, where turmeric is a national healing plant, are much less frequent than in the Western world. The authors of one of these studies ascribe this positive result to the nightly ingestion of a Temoe Lawa tea made out of turmeric. It is not only such studies, but also individual examinations of humans and animals that confirm the stimulation of bile production and release through turmeric: experiments have shown that people who ingested 3 grams of turmeric had a two- to threefold increase in their bile production.

The enzymes in ginger also enhance digestion, especially the amylases and protease, which break down starches and proteins. They ensure that food is more easily digested and does not weigh so heavily in the stomach. The ginger enzymes become active even before the food is eaten. They tenderize meat during preparation in the kitchen (but more about this is in the recipe section).

How to use ginger, turmeric, cardamom, and galangal: Add fresh or dried spices often and generously to dishes, or prepare a cup of tea with them and drink it before the meal. This facilitates digestion. For digestive problems, pour 1 cup of water over 1 teaspoon powdered dried ginger and let it steep for 5 to 10 minutes while keeping the cup covered. Pour through a strainer and drink before the meal.

It is unusual to prepare tea out of turmeric alone, but in combination with other bile active spices it can be used to prepare an effective gallbladder tea. Here is an example of such a tea:

Java turmeric	20 parts
dandelions with roots	20 parts
peppermint leaves	20 parts
yarrow leaves	20 parts
cardamom seeds	20 parts

Mix the ingredients and make a tea with the ratio of 1 cup of hot water to 3 teaspoons of the mixture. Steep for 10 minutes, then strain the liquid through a sieve. Drink the tea three times a day.

Alternately, we recommend taking 1/2 gram powdered turmeric three or four times a day.

Warning: If you have gallstones you should not consume large amounts of ginger and turmeric without consulting your doctor. Smaller amounts used for seasoning foods do not pose any threat.

GINGER FOR STOMACH ULCERS

A medical saying holds true for ulcers: no hurry, no curry, no worry. Ginger, however, seems to be an exception to the rule. As paradoxical as this may sound, during animal testing it was shown that some ingredients of ginger could prevent stress-related damage to the stomach's mucous membrane. Researchers ascribe this effect in part to the volatile oils. But certain spicy constituents also protect against ulcers.

How to use ginger: Those with sensitive stomachs should mix fresh ginger with their food only shortly before serving, instead of cooking the ginger with the food. This ensures that the ginger's volatile oils remain intact, and that the gingerol will not have transformed into the spicier shogaol.

CARDAMOM FOR HEARTBURN

Those who suffer from acid indigestion should consult a doctor, since this can be a symptom of serious illnesses. In other cases the problem can be alleviated by some simple measures:

35

- eat mostly high-protein, low-fat foods
- eat several small meals a day, instead of three large meals
- reduce excess body weight
- avoid tight clothing
- avoid nicotine, coffee, and alcohol

Instead of drinking coffee or black tea, drink one cup of the following several times a day:

cardamom seeds	40 parts
cumin seeds	30 parts
fennel seeds	30 parts

Crush 2 teaspoons of this seed mixture, then pour hot water over it and let the mixture sit covered for 10 minutes. Drink it warm, but not hot, in small sips during or after meals.

GINGER, CARDAMOM, AND GALANGAL AGAINST FLATULENCE

Ginger and galangal turn into "hot sweepers" in the intestine. They destroy many harmful bacteria and parasites and regulate the balance of healthy intestinal flora. Laboratory studies have shown that spicy constituents and volatile oils slow down the reproduction of undesirable bacteria in the large intestine, those that live off undigested carbohydrates. The bacterial decomposition of the hard-to-digest remains of, for example, legumes often lead to flatulence. Ginger and galangal will put an end to this. Furthermore, ginger encourages the growth of acidopholus bacteria, which help with the digestion. Acidopholus bacteria break carbohydrates down into simple sugars without creating gases.

The effectiveness of cardamom against flatulence can also be traced back to its volatile oils. Much like cumin and fennel, cardamom helps in relaxing the muscles in the intestine and thus helps the release of intestinal gases. Moreover, volatile oils have a slightly antibacterial effect.

How to use ginger, galangal, and cardamom:
Foods that are most likely to cause flatulence, such as cabbage, legumes, and onions, should be thoroughly seasoned with these three spice lilies. However, add these spices only toward the end of cooking, otherwise a large part of the volatile oils will be lost.

If these spices are not appropriate for the flavor of your meal, a tasty tea can also be prepared from cardamom seeds. You can make the tea entirely out of cardamom seeds, which have to be crushed just before steeping, or in combination with equal parts of fennel, and/or cumin seeds. Two teaspoons of this mixture should be freshly ground, the better to release the volatile oils. Mortar and pestle are best suited for this job, but those who do not have a mortar and pestle can simply place the ingredients on a steady surface and crush them with the back of a wooden spoon. It is important to crush only the amount needed immediately, as the seed shells provide the best protection for keeping the volatile oils intact. Once the seeds are crushed, the oils rapidly lose their quality.

CARDAMOM FOR FRESH BREATH

Especially after the consumption of onions or garlic, one's breath can develop an unpleasant odor. Meat and fish can cause an unpleasant taste in the mouth as well. Meat in particular gets stuck in the spaces between the teeth and starts to rot. It is a good idea to brush your teeth carefully after such meals, or bad breath may cause others to avoid you. Mouth sprays are not particularly effective for this problem. Consistently good oral hygiene, especially flossing, is the best remedy.

Bad breath, however, does not only occur after meals, among some people it is caused by a lack of saliva or by insufficient digestion of meals. When insufficient saliva is the problem it helps to drink a lot and to eat a candy or a snack several times a day to stimulate salivation. As was discussed in the previous chapter, spices such as ginger and galangal stimulate the digestion.

Warning: In cases of chronic heartburn or reflux of stomach acid, a doctor should be consulted.

How to use cardamom: Garlic odors and bad breath can be fought by chewing cardamom seeds. The volatile oils discourage growth of bacteria in the mouth and make for fresh breath. This aromatic seed is also beneficial for fighting infections of the mouth's mucous membrane.

Nausea and Vomiting— Natural Prevention with Ginger

SEASICKNESS

When the sea gets rough many travelers get seasick. People suddenly turn quiet and pale, with cold sweat appearing on their foreheads. If the motion persists, they vomit. This response is not unusual and happens even to experienced sailors.

Doctors have been researching the origins of seasickness for a long time. Napoleon's personal doctor believed he had found the cure for motion sickness. He believed that the symptoms were caused by the brain mass flowing back and forth. He thus believed that young and intelligent people, who have large and soft brains, were most affected by motion sickness. As a cure, he recommended that the afflicted tie bands tightly around their foreheads.

Although this remedy provided little relief for the afflicted, doctors today have a more precise idea of what causes motion sickness. They believe that the symptoms of seasickness are caused not by an actual sickness, but rather by the effects of unusual motions on the vestibular system, the organs of balance in the inner ear. Motions that cause sickness exceed the limits that the vestibular system can report accurately to the brain. When the vestibular system reports false information to the brain, that information conflicts with the information reported by the eyes and other sense organs. On a rolling and pitching boat, for example, the vestibular system might report that the body is moving upward while the eyes report that the body is moving downward.

But why should this conflicting information cause nausea and vomiting? Research has shown that the vestibular system, besides regulating balance, also functions as part of the body's mechanism for detecting poisons. When certain poisons are present in the blood, the vestibular system malfunctions and reports false information. The brain responds to this information by causing vomiting in order to empty any remaining poison from the stomach. Research suggests that motion sickness occurs when the brain misinterprets the false information caused by excessive motion, interpreting it as a sign of poisoning instead.

When seasickness is a possibility, it is important to take preventive measures. Once nausea has arisen, any remedies are usually too late to be of much help. Here are some tips for sea travel:

- If you have the choice between a motorboat and a sailboat of the same size, take the sailboat. It is easier to get sick on a motorboat. While a sailboat is tilted in the water, its movement around its long axis, the rolling movement, is dampened by the stabilizing effects of sail and keel.

- Try to stay near the point of rotation of the ship, at the cross of the long and the short axes. This is where the boat moves the least. Stay above deck, keep your head steady, and try to focus on the horizon. It is the only stable optical object of comparison.

- If possible, take the rudder yourself. The concentration on the horizon and the distraction of steering are ideal preventive measures. If all methods fail, it is better to lie down and try to sleep.

- You should always avoid alcohol, since it influences your balance, which can be a problem even on land.

A small consolation for those who have booked a boat trip of several days' duration: our balance perception gradually gets used to the movements on a boat and stops rebelling. The adjustment process takes less time if you get plenty of sleep before leaving. But the adjustment process only works on boats of comparable size, thus it is better not to switch from a large boat to a small boat or vice versa. Charles Darwin observed in his journals that seamen who had gotten used to the movements of a large ship would get seasick in a rowboat.

CARSICKNESS

Passengers can experience motion sickness when riding in cars too, for example when the driver alternately slows down and accelerates for turns, or when the passenger turns, lifts, or lowers the head on a winding road. But the driver does not get sick on even the most winding roads because his eyes and his body and his concentration follow the curves as he drives. The movement that is registered by his vestibular system is confirmed by his other sensory organs, for example his eyes.

A passenger experiences the motion differently, especially if he is reading in the car or sitting in the backseat. While the balance organ in the ear reports movements, the eye reports a seemingly steady picture. These conflicting reports confuse the brain, and it responds with nausea. As with seasickness, the best defense against carsickness is to take preventive measures. Here are some tips for avoiding carsickness:

- Sit in front if possible.
- Children riding in the back are sick less frequently if they sit high up in their seats and have an unobstructed view of the outside.

- In buses the seats up in front, ideally just be-hind the front axle, are best.
- In no case should you read on a curvy road.

Acupressure bands, another aid against motion sickness, come from traditional Chinese medicine. An elastic wristband with a button on it is attached to the wrist in such a way that the button pushes against the inside of the wrist on a specific acupressure point that relieves nausea. Of course, the Chinese have been aware of the effectiveness of ginger in fighting motion sickness for centuries as well.

WITH GINGER ON BOARD, NAUSEA DISAPPEARS

As Chinese travelers from the fifth century report, the great Chinese seafarers of earlier times took ginger on board to ward off seasickness. Once planted, the bulb quickly begins to sprout, sending up fresh green shoots that are tender and have a mild taste. To fight nausea, the sailors simply chewed these shoots.

Now modern medicine has confirmed ginger's effectiveness. Comparative studies have also shown that ginger fights nausea just as well as chemical substances do. In one study, dried ground ginger performed even better than dimenhydrinate, which was used for comparison. Dimenhydrinate is a synthetic substance included in most travel medications. It is the spicy constituents in ginger that are believed to be effective against motion sickness. In laboratory experiments gingerol as well as shogaol offered effective protection against vomiting.

It is not clear exactly how these substances work. They might have some influence on the central nervous system, but the spicy constituents mainly calm the digestive tract. They relax muscles and relieve cramps there as well as relaxing the blood vessels of the stomach. Circulation to the stomach is thus increased, its digestive activity stimulated, and tensions alleviated. Thus ginger not only alleviates motion sickness but relieves nausea resulting from medication or simple indigestion caused by overeating.

In contrast to the synthetic substances for nausea, which are antihistamines, ginger preparations do not cause drowsiness. The distorted vision that is often caused by antihistamines is not a problem with ginger either. In general, by taking ginger instead of commercial travel medications, one can avoid the long list of side effects that come with the commercial preparations.

How to use ginger: Take two to four capsules of powdered ginger, 250 milligrams each, about half an hour before the beginning of the journey, and take one more every four hours. For those who do not find it unpleasant, chewing fresh ginger is recommended as well.

STUDIES WITH GINGER

Numerous studies have researched the effects of ginger on motion sickness. One study was done with eighty young seamen between the ages of sixteen and nineteen. Before sailing, each received either 1 gram ginger powder or a placebo. The results showed that compared with the placebo group, the group that received the ginger experienced significantly fewer cases of cold sweat, dizziness, and nausea.

In a different study on a cruise ship, sixty participants between the ages of ten and seventy-seven were tested for the effects of ginger. One group took 500 milligrams ginger powder every four hours, while the other participants received 100 milligrams of dimenhydrinate. In this study, ginger prevented travel sickness as well as the synthetic medication, while causing fewer side effects.

Similar results were obtained by a larger study that involved fifteen hundred tourists on a safari. The participants took 500 milligrams ginger powder every four hours or alternatively various other medications for nausea. Here too, ginger proved equal to other medications.

In yet another study, thirty-six students with severe cases of motion sickness underwent an experiment involving a rotating chair that induced nausea among the participants. Before the test, the participants received 1 gram ginger powder, or 100 milligrams dimenhydrinate, or a placebo. Those students who had ingested the ginger lasted significantly longer on the chair than those who had taken the medication or the placebo. In this study, ginger proved superior to the synthetic medication.

But not all studies attest to the effectiveness of ginger. Some studies have not been able to demonstrate the effectiveness of ginger. Negative results could be attributed to the varying quality of the ginger preparations used, as well as to the widely varying conditions of the experiments.

MORNING SICKNESS

Most women experience at least some nausea in the mornings during the first months of their pregnancy; many vomit frequently. Usually morning sickness is not a cause for worry as it is simply a normal bodily reaction to the hormones produced during pregnancy. If the patient is vomiting very frequently though, the resulting loss of liquids and electrolytes can cause problems. She should consult with her doctor about this. Sometimes intravenous treatment in a hospital will be necessary to restore normal fluid levels. Aside from the hormonal changes, stress factors such as problems with a partner or financial troubles can exacerbate morning sickness as well.

The medical treatment of morning sickness poses problems, as the fetus will be affected by the medication as well. That is why any medication has to be considered very carefully during a pregnancy. Before resorting to prescription medications, try these tips for relieving morning sickness:

- Take several small meals throughout the day instead of three large ones, the first one preferably while you are still in bed. You can put some cookies or crackers next to your bed the night before.
- Drink a cup of herbal tea before getting up. Lemon balm, chamomile, or peppermint would be good choices. (You can prepare these teas the night before and keep them warm in a thermos.)
- The ingestion of vitamin B6 in amounts between 160 to 600 milligrams per day has proved beneficial for many women.

GINGER FOR MORNING SICKNESS

Since ginger is so good for relieving nausea in general, it made sense to research its effectiveness for morning sickness. To this end, thirty women in the seventh through the seventeenth week of pregnancy took 250 milligrams ginger per day for four days, followed by two days without medication. After that the women received a placebo for four days. The patients receiving ginger felt much better and experienced less nausea. The treatment had no effect on the fetus.

The FDA considers ginger capsules to be safe and

free from risks. Ginger has no known pharmaceutical effects on the fetus. Only in Germany has there been hesitation in recommending ginger for morning sickness, not because ginger has any proven negative effects but simply because they feel more studies should be done on the effects of ginger on the embryo.

OTHER TYPES OF NAUSEA

As a reaction to anesthesia, nausea and vomiting frequently occur after surgery. That is why the effectiveness of ginger has also been tested in connection with surgery anesthetics. For both minor and major surgical procedures, patients received 1 gram of ginger before the anesthesia. In both studies, ginger proved to be very effective.

Many medications also cause nausea, especially medications used in the treatment of cancer. One study comparing ginger with a placebo showed that ginger is effective for combatting nausea here as well.

Ginger and Turmeric—
Providing Strength for the
Heart and Blood Vessels

Heart and circulation problems are among the most common causes of death in the United States. Doctors call heart attacks and strokes "civilization diseases," but Americans and Europeans are not the only civilized peoples of this world. In other highly industrialized and technologically advanced countries, such as Japan, these diseases are far less prevalent. It is obvious that the difference between Eastern and Western diets has a big influence on the circulatory system. The Asian diet, which is rich in fish and vegetables, is certainly more "heart healthy." Perhaps ginger and turmeric, both used frequently in Asian cooking, play a small role in preventing heart and circulatory diseases. The ingredients of both plants affect the heart, the circulation, and especially the blood itself.

INFLUENCE ON THE CHOLESTEROL LEVEL

An elevated cholesterol level is among the risk factors for arteriosclerosis. When fatty streaks of excess cholesterol are deposited on blood vessel walls, the vessels become harder, narrower, and less flexible. In worst-case scenarios, the fatty deposits enlarge and thicken to form rough-edged plaques that irritate the smooth lining of the arteries, causing cells to die and scars to form. Thus the flow of blood is constricted, the transport of oxygen and nutrients to the various organs is impeded, and waste products are not carried off by the blood as effectively. The rough surface of the arteries can cause a thrombus, or blood clot, to form on the arterial wall. A thrombus can suddenly block circulation in a given artery. The complete blockage of an artery supplying the heart or the brain results in a heart attack or a stroke, respectively.

The clogging of arteries is a gradual process that cannot be reversed. Thus prevention becomes very important. The best means of prevention is to reduce the consumption of animal fats. Eating more garlic is recommended too, as garlic is well known for its ability to lower cholesterol levels. But many people avoid garlic because of its strong smell, fearing bad breath or an unpleasant body odor if they consume it in large quantities.

For those who avoid garlic but still want to do something positive for their cholesterol levels, science has promising news: turmeric and ginger may provide an effective alternative. Results of experiments performed on laboratory rats show that turmeric and ginger can slow the elevation of cholesterol levels even with a cholesterol rich diet. This is because their ingredients inhibit the absorption of cholesterol into the bloodstream and facilitate the excretion of cholesterol as well.

But before you depend on ginger to lower your blood cholesterol level, you should wait for the results from further studies. It has not yet been demonstrated that the results obtained from animal testing can be applied to humans. Eating unlimited animal fats without regrets will not be possible, even with ginger and turmeric. But if you are going to consume animal fats, you should at least do it with the right spices.

AS EFFECTIVE AS ASPIRIN?

Ginger and turmeric have other traits in common with garlic besides their effects on cholesterol levels. All three of these spices also improve the consistency of the blood. Laboratory experiments have shown that ginger and turmeric contain ingredients that inhibit the production of the cyclooxygenase (COX) enzymes that synthesize prostaglandins in our bodies. Prostaglandins are fatty acids with hormonelike properties. As prostaglandins encourage the coagulation of the blood, reducing their levels acts to thin the blood, thus preventing the blood clots that can lead to heart attack or stroke.

This is the same mechanism as that activated by aspirin. Aspirin, with the active ingredient acetylsalicylic acid, is one of the most important medications used today in the prevention of strokes and heart attacks.

Ginger and turmeric are not going to take this important role away from aspirin. Nonetheless, something that was discovered in laboratory experiments has been confirmed by a small study in India using ginger on healthy men. The men ate 100 grams of butter every day for seven days. This was followed by seven days during which half of the men ingested 5 grams of dried ginger per day with their food, while the other half did not. Scientists monitored the effects of ginger on the composition of the blood. They paid particular attention to the stickiness of the blood platelets (red blood cells)—that is, their tendency to clump together and form clots. Clotting was reduced significantly in the group that had ingested the ginger. Similar results were shown for women who received fresh ginger. Here, too, blood clotting was significantly lower in the group that ingested ginger than in the placebo group. Studies testing smaller doses of ginger were less successful.

IT WARMS THE HEART

The ingestion of ginger immediately produces a sensation of cozy warmth as the active ingredients spread throughout the body. In traditional Chinese medicine, ginger is regarded as a plant that produces inner warmth and opens up new paths of energy. While Western scientists are not quite as poetic, they do confirm that ginger has a stimulating effect on the heart muscle and thus strengthens the heart. A strong heart muscle can pump more blood per contraction into the surrounding blood vessels. This allows the heart to slow down, switching from many weak beats per minute to a few strong ones. In this way, the heart operates much more economically.

The strong heartbeats improve circulation throughout the body and the body's supply of oxygen and nutrients. The better blood transport benefits blood pressure levels as well. With regular consumption of ginger, a slight lowering of blood pressure has been observed, because ginger relaxes and dilates the blood vessels. This further reduces stress on the heart.

How to use ginger: Those that have problems getting up in the mornings and are often cold during the day can benefit greatly from ginger's warming and stimulating properties. Ginger cereal for breakfast gets you in shape for the day and a ginger soup makes a warming snack.

A morning massage with about 4 percent volatile ginger oil dissolved in jojoba oil or a moisturizing lotion also stimulates the circulation. Undiluted ginger oil, however, should not be used as it could cause skin irritations.

HOT AND COLD AT THE SAME TIME

Though we might expect that they would only worsen the heat, hot beverages and spicy foods are frequently consumed in tropical climates. In fact the spicy constituents in ginger, gingerol and shogaol, stimulate warmth receptors and cause a pleasant warm feeling in stomach and intestines, which in turn opens the pores and stimulates the sweat glands. The evaporation of the sweat from the skin has a cooling effect on the body.

Natural Relief from
Arthritis and Joint Pain

Arthritis is an ailment with many faces. The best known and most common type is chronic osteo-arthrosis, a gradual degenerative condition in which the primary cause of pain is the degeneration of the layer of joint cartilage that cushions the juncture of one bone with another. Joints may stiffen into a bent position, and range of motion is diminished. Later, fluid may build up in the joint, causing it to swell and distort, which stretches connecting liga-ments, destabilizing the joint and producing pain. Arthritic symptoms can also be caused by rheuma-toid arthritis, an autoimmune disease in which im-mune cells mistakenly attack collagen (the chief building material of skin, cartilage, tendons, and ligaments), producing inflammatory chemicals in the joint fluid that degrade cartilage and bone. Rheumatoid arthritis can affect the skin and inter-nal organs as well, instigating conditions such as psoriasis and Crohn's disease.

Currently, chronic arthritis cannot be healed; the goal of treatment is merely to slow down the process of degeneration, to alleviate inflammation, and to com-bat pain. The most common family of medications used for arthritic pain relief are the non-steroidal anti-inflammatory drugs (NSAIDs), including diclofenac, indomethacin, ibuprofen, and acetylsalicylic acid (aspirin). The NSAIDs are effective blockers of both the mechanical pain of osteoarthritis and the inflammatory pain of rheumatoid arthritis. But especially at the high doses required to control arthritic pain, these medications have serious gastric side effects, inhibiting the formation of the stomach's protective mucous membrane, which can result in erosion of the stomach lining. Researchers are constantly looking for alternative treatments for controlling the pain of arthritis without negative side effects.

Of course, in addition to synthetic drugs, researchers look into natural plant derivatives for possible treatments. A balsamic resin derived from Indian frankincense *(Boswellia serrata)* showed early promise. Like ginger, frankincense is a traditional ayurvedic medicine. The main active ingredients of frankincense are two boswellic acids that have been shown to be effective anti-inflammatory agents. The boswellic acids inhibit the production of leukotrienes, fatty acids in the blood that act as pain mediators, encouraging the inflammatory cascade reactions of escalating pain and inflammation set off by an overactive autoimmune system. Promising study results report that pain, swelling, and morning stiffness were all reduced significantly among arthritis patients taking frankincense. In comparison to the record of side effects for the usual rheumatic medicines, only a few mild side effects were recorded for frankincense.

GINGER AND TURMERIC
IN RHEUMATIC THERAPY

Ginger and turmeric have been used to treat infectious diseases in the Orient for millennia. These practical applications have been researched more closely in recent years. In the course of researching these plants, their counteracting effects on the cox enzymes have been reaffirmed. Remember that these enzymes initiate the formation of prostaglandins in the blood. Besides acting to thicken the blood, increasing the risk of strokes, prostaglandins also act as pain mediators in the same way that leukotrienes do, encouraging painful inflammatory cascade reactions.

In animal testing, ginger and turmeric extracts have clearly shown their effectiveness in slowing inflammation and lowering fevers. This can be confirmed especially for the isolated spicy constituents of ginger, 6-gingerol and 6-shogaol. In this case the shogaol proved superior to the gingerol. Animal testing has also shown that the effects of ginger and turmeric extracts can even be compared favorably to prescription arthritis medications. This result inspires hope, but unfortunately can not simply be transferred to humans, especially since the extracts were injected into the research animals. How completely these extracts would be absorbed by the body when eating meals containing ginger and turmeric and how effective they would be in treating human symptoms are questions that have not been studied sufficiently.

For ginger, though, the results of small studies in Denmark have been published that describe its effects on humans suffering from arthritis. Its effectiveness was tested on a small group of seven patients between the ages of fifty and sixty-seven. These men and women all suffered from chronic joint pain. All patients were taking standard NSAIDs to manage the pain. Some patients had been treated with cortisone or gold salts as well. These medications brought about some temporary relief, but the patients were not freed of the symptoms.

One patient, a fifty-year-old Asian male, ingested 5 grams of fresh ginger as soon as he experienced symptoms. He boiled the ginger briefly before taking it. Within thirty days of starting this therapy, pain and signs of inflammation had diminished substantially. After three months of ginger therapy, the pain and swelling was almost gone. The man was able to work once again as a car mechanic. He has continued ginger therapy for ten years now without suffering a relapse.

The other six patients also started by ingesting 5 grams fresh ginger, or 1/2 to 1 gram ginger powder. Before beginning the therapy they had not taken cortisone or gold salts for at least three months. The patients had continued taking their pain-relieving medicine. When they ingested the ginger their symptoms diminished markedly, enabling them to use less synthetic medication. After three months all patients reported that the pain and swelling had diminished, and that the flexibility of their joints had increased. None of the patients experienced any side effects throughout the therapy. Patients reported feeling better in general and were able to be more active.

In another survey, fifty-six patients with different types of arthritis took varying amounts of ginger. Most patients reported substantial improvement in their conditions. Some were entirely freed of the symptoms. The patients had previously taken synthetic arthritis medication, but they had not experienced sufficient relief of their symptoms, or the relief had come only with unacceptable side effects. With the additional ingestion of ginger, joint flexibility increased among 75 percent of the participants. They experienced less pain, and swelling diminished.

While these observations of patients did not meet all the requirements of a double-blind scientific study, the reported results do warrant further scientific investigation in this area.

At an arthritis congress in Singapore in 1997, a Danish study was presented in which ginger was tested in comparison to a placebo and to a synthetic arthritis medicine. The study compared the pain-reducing characteristics of the three substances, as well as the side effects experienced. This study was double-blind, meaning that neither the doctors nor the patients knew which of the three capsules they were administering or receiving. Fifty-six patients participated in this study for six weeks.

The results showed that, while ginger was clearly superior to the placebo, it could not match the effectiveness of the synthetic medication. Both substances exhibited the best results toward the end of the six-week period.

In the spring of 1998 a new study was initiated in Germany that compares the effectiveness of varying dosages of ginger powder. This study, which is taking place in Berlin, involves 100 participants with mild to medium cases of arthritis. At first the patients received 500 milligrams of ginger powder, in capsule form, two times daily. If no improvement was recorded after two weeks, the dosage was increased to 500 milligrams three times a day. Although the results of this study are not yet available, the initial reports are encouraging.

We are not suggesting that you rely on ginger in place of scientific medical treatment, but anecdotal evidence does suggest that the plant can bring noticeable relief from arthritic symptoms. A supplemental ginger therapy can often reduce the amount of synthetic medication required to control symptoms, thus also reducing their side effects. Several natural healing clinics are already using ginger powder in capsules for the treatment of arthritis.

How to use ginger: Finely chop or grind 5 grams of fresh ginger and mix in with the food. Those who do not enjoy spicy food should boil the ginger briefly. The active ingredients do not suffer from this. On the contrary, the shogaol, which is made available by boiling, is supposed to be even more effective against inflammation than the spicy constituents available in raw ginger.

Those who do not want to cook with ginger on a daily basis can also take ginger in capsules. So far, no concrete dosage for arthritic symptoms is available.

Other Healing Applications for the Spice Lilies

Much of the potential of the ginger family has not yet been researched. Practical experience as well as scientific laboratories offer many interesting leads as to possible healing effects, many of which need further investigation. Some of these will be presented briefly in the following pages.

GINGER FOR EXHAUSTION

Tired, exhausted, burnt out—with the hectic pace of life these days who hasn't experienced these symptoms? Nature offers something to combat exhaustion—the warm ginger compress. To make the compress, mix ginger powder with warm water and apply to the spine. The patient should lie on his or her stomach in a comfortable place. After applying the ginger paste, cover the spine with a cloth, and then the whole back with another cloth. The stimulating effect of ginger on the circulation, which was discussed in detail in the section "Ginger and Turmeric—Providing Strength for the Heart and Blood Vessels," stimulates the metabolism and the patient will soon be reenergized.

The immune system is activated by ginger as well. With improved circulation, the immune cells can be transported more quickly throughout the body, and the cells fight disease more efficiently as well. Laboratory experiments have researched the direct influence of ginger on human immune cells and have shown that ginger extract causes cells to produce more defensive substances.

GINGER FOR INFLUENZA

Fever is a healthy bodily reaction in response to invasion by infectious substances. It is triggered by the immune system when the immune cells encounter infectious substances in the bloodstream. They report their findings to the brain, which in turn increases the body temperature to help destroy the invaders.

To fight the infection, the body's normal temperature of 98.6°F needs to increase. In order to accomplish the increase, the blood vessels in the skin contract so as to avoid losing body heat, producing the so-called goose bumps. Moreover, the muscles start to shake in order to generate heat. These two measures increase the temperature so that we register a fever.

After the infectious substances have been successfully destroyed, the temperature returns to normal. In order to lower the body temperature, the pores in the skin open up and the body starts to sweat. The evaporation of sweat from the skin brings the body temperature down.

In Western alternative medicine, fevers are broken with sweat-inducing plants such as elder petals and linden petals. Traditional Chinese medicine uses ginger for chills associated with fever, since it warms the body from the inside and then supports natural sweating.

But there is another reason why ginger and turmeric can be used in the latter phases of a fever. As mentioned earlier, the two act in a way similar to acetylsalicylic acid in combating rheumatic infections and the clotting of blood platelets. Much like aspirin, these plants prevent the formation of prostaglandin. Prostaglandin also plays a role in fevers, which is why aspirin has the capacity to lower a fever. Thus it is conceivable that ginger and turmeric can lower an increased temperature the natural way. This theory has been confirmed in animal testing.

How to use ginger: When you feel a flu and a fever coming on, stay in bed and drink one cup of hot ginger tea several times a day. Pour boiling water over 1 teaspoon dried ginger and let the tea sit for 5 to 10 minutes. Strain it through a sieve afterward. For more tasty ginger tea recipes, consult the recipe section later in this book.

CARDAMOM TO ALLEVIATE A COUGH

Cardamom tea has made a name for itself as an expectorant. It helps resolve a persistent dry cough with little phlegm. Its volatile oils cause more fluids to be excreted so that the phlegm can be coughed up more easily. The volatile oil also increases the activity of the hairs of the bronchioles, which act to loosen the phlegm. Moreover, cardamom oil, like most volatile oils, has an antibacterial effect (but more about this later on).

How to use cardamom: An expectorant tea made from cardamom seeds can be prepared like this— pour hot water over 2 teaspoons crushed seeds, then pour through a sieve. Drink several warm cups of this tea a day.

GINGER TO SUPPRESS A COUGH

Ginger is supposed to be effective for suppressing a persistent cough. Animal testing has shown that the spicy constituent shogaol blocks the cough reflex in the cough center of the central nervous system. Ginger tea should be considered in cases of a severe cough without any phlegm. At night as well, when constant coughing prevents rest, ginger tea can be used to suppress the cough.

EFFECTS ON BACTERIA, VIRUSES, AND OTHER INTRUDERS

In laboratories, ginger, turmeric, and cardamom have proven effective in slowing the growth of numerous bacteria. In one study, turmeric demonstrated effectiveness against a strain of bacteria that causes gallbladder infections. In test tube trials cardamom even impaired herpes viruses. To what degree these results can be translated into practice has not yet been examined. However, turmeric is often used in everyday life to treat skin ailments because of its effects against infections and bacteria. And turmeric has also provided effective protection against insect pests in stored grains, for example in rice or wheat.

Ginger has also exhibited another interesting effect, which is also applied in praxis. The volatile oils gingerol and shogaol kill some parasites, for example the schistosomes, tropical parasitic worms that invade the bloodstream, causing the often deadly disease schistosomiasis or bilharzia. This serious disease causes blood loss and tissue damage.

EFFECTIVE FOR MIGRAINES

Many people suffer from this particularly debilitating type of headache. Migraine headaches occur unilaterally—that is, the pain is only on one side of the head—and are often accompanied by nausea, dizziness, vomiting, and visual disturbances. They usually do not last more than twenty-four hours, but migraine sufferers tend to have recurring attacks. Sometimes migraines are linked to a woman's hormonal reproductive cycle, appearing along with ovulation or menstruation. There is no known cure, but there are innumerable suggestions, both good and bad, as to how to get rid of a migraine or how to prevent one from occurring.

In ayurvedic medicine, ginger is successfully used to treat migraines. Ginger researchers are now proposing that migraine sufferers should take ginger on a preventive basis. One research team describes the case of a forty-two-year-old woman who took between 1.5 and 2 grams ginger for three to four days. She then further integrated ginger into her diet. She noticed that the frequency of her migraines decreased significantly.

In popular medicine, turmeric is also used for headaches. Mix turmeric powder into Vaseline to make a paste and apply to the face, especially the forehead and temples. But be careful; yellow spots may remain on the skin. They will disappear within a few days.

PROTECTION FOR THE CELLS

Turmeric and ginger also act as antioxidants, chemical compounds that block the effects of oxidation. Oxidation is a chemical reaction in which a substance loses electrons when combining with oxygen. Unstable molecules called free radicals are produced by oxidation. Scientists believe free radicals play a role in the aging process as well as in a number of diseases, such as arteriosclerosis, Alzheimer's disease, and cancer. They are damaging to the body because they can take electrons away from almost any nearby molecule to replace their own lost electrons, eroding cells or causing changes in genes in the process.

Cells create free radicals when oxygen combines with food molecules to produce energy. Their production can be triggered by radiation, cigarette smoke, and air pollution as well. So it is important to block the negative effects of free radicals by including antioxidants in your diet. Vitamins C and E and the plant chemicals known as carotinoids and flavinoids are good antioxidants. They can be found in fruits and vegetables, particularly those that are dark green or deep yellow. And now turmeric and ginger are considered to neutralize free radicals as well.

SUPPORT FOR THE LIVER

Almost everything we eat and drink is channeled through the liver. The liver is the largest metabolic organ in the human body. It plays a key role in breaking down fats to make their nutrients available to the body. The liver is also the largest gland in the body. It produces almost one quart of bile every day, which is necessary for fat digestion. The liver also cleanses the blood, filtering out toxins and directing them to the kidneys for excretion. The liver can withstand these high demands if it is not damaged by viruses or toxins, such as excessive alcohol consumption.

In the practice of natural healing the fruits of the milk thistle have the largest significance for liver ailments. They offer a double protection: their ingredients change the liver cells in such a way that no toxins can enter, and they also improve the organ's capacity to regenerate by stimulating the creation of new liver cells. Milk thistle preparations thus act preventively when toxins threaten a healthy liver as well as regeneratively in the acute stages of liver damage.

Turmeric and ginger also support the liver. Liver cells bred in laboratories showed that the spicy constituents of the two plants were able to protect the cells from the destructive effects of a toxic solvent. A further study compared the relative effects of several different spicy constituents. This study showed that gingerol was more effective than shogaol for protecting the liver. Complete research to support this thesis is still in its early stages though.

THIN WITH GINGER?

Each boom attracts clever entrepreneurs that are looking to make a quick buck without any serious commitment to the customer. Those who long to lose weight often prove to be easy marks for unscrupulous businessmen. Capsules with ginger and pineapple that are supposed to reduce excess weight have hit the market recently. The bitter constituents of ginger and so-called protein-splitting enzymes are supposed to be responsible for this effect. Do not be fooled! Ginger actually tends to stimulate the appetite and would thus encourage weight gain rather than weight loss. It is certainly true that food is digested better because of the ginger-pineapple capsules, but you will keep

RAW OR COOKED?

How should one handle spices to profit the most from their healthy ingredients? There is no consistent strategy for this, since different ingredients have different effects. During cooking the volatile oils disappear, which is why cardamom should only be added toward the end of cooking. The enzymes in ginger and other bioactive substances are also destroyed during cooking. However, in ginger, cooking produces the spicy constituents gingerol and shogaol, which are the effective ingredients for treating some conditions. How exactly these substances act in the body can only be speculated about at this point in time. For the medical studies on ginger, turmeric, and galangal, the dried and freshly powdered roots were used, whereas for cardamom the dried seeds were used. Industrially processed ginger, in ginger ale or gingersnaps for example, does not have much to offer in the way of health benefits.

your weight unless you eat significantly fewer calories, especially in the form of fat. Those who follow this guideline will lose weight with or without ginger.

The Spice Lilies Have Few Undesirable Side Effects

"The dosage is the key." This wise sentence from the well-known doctor Paracelsus applies to herbal medicine as well as conventional medicine. Moderate dosage makes sense especially when one considers that plants usually produce their active ingredients to deter animals from eating them. In normal doses, ginger, turmeric, cardamom, and galangal are not toxic but are safe, healing substances. Almost no side effects have been reported. Only in very rare cases do allergies arise to some of the ingredients. If very large amounts are consumed before going to bed, some reports have suggested that ginger affects dreams.

If volatile oils or extracts are used externally for massages, some people with very sensitive skin may experience irritations. Often the ingredients responsible for the irritation are the same ones that stimulate circulation, which is exactly what is desired. To avoid irritation, volatile oils should not be applied to the skin in their pure forms; rather, they should be diluted at a ratio of 1:10 with vegetable oils such as Jojoba oil or almond oil. Then skin irritations will no longer occur.

WHO SHOULD BE CAREFUL
WHEN USING GINGER AS A MEDICINE?

- Since ginger and turmeric stimulate the production of bile, which is stored in the gallbladder, patients with gallstones should consult their doctors before taking larger quantities (more than 1 gram of powder per day) of ginger or turmeric.

- So far there have not been sufficient studies on the possible adverse effects of ginger taken for morning sickness. Thus you should consult your doctor here too.

- Patients who take medication against the clotting of blood platelets, for example acetylsalicylic acid (aspirin), or ticlopidine (Ticlid) should consult a doctor before taking large quantities of ginger and turmeric.

If the spice lilies are merely used as spices for cooking, there is no reason to worry, even in the three situations mentioned above.

4

Healthy Cooking
with the
Ginger Family

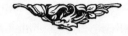

HEALTHY COOKING is experiencing a boom as the scientific evidence mounts linking excessive consumption of fats, salt, and processed foods to the rise in obesity, cancer, heart attacks, and strokes. Numerous cookbooks, diet guides, and health books speak to the search for the ideal diet. They all contain hints as to what is healthy, and what is not. But the number of guides has now become a jungle, in which you will encounter both reasonable and absurd suggestions. The consumer is faced with the problem of choosing those tips most applicable to his or her own situation. How can one distinguish between the good advice and the bad?

When judging a diet or health regimen, a few questions will often suffice. How fanatically rigid is the program? Are the ideas presented with a sense of humor? Is there an acceptance of the enjoyment principle? How realistic would it be to follow the suggestions for a long time? How radical are the suggestions? Which foods does the diet recommend refraining from, and why? Are these foods a core part of your current diet? How unhappy would you be if you had to forego them?

Those who want to change their diets face a hard task. Many programs are so restrictive that any person who enjoys living cannot abide by them for long. If you tell yourself to eat no meat, no fat, no sugar, no alcohol, no coffee, no black tea, no white flour, and you substitute a strict regimen of warm water, herbal teas, steamed vegetables, rice, whole wheat bread, and raw vegetables for the forbidden foods, in the long run you will not feel satisfied. One day you will find yourself sneaking back into the nearest steak house to eat something "real" for a change. Or you'll go to your favorite bakery and order that piece of pie you've been dreaming about for weeks.

What good are dietary rules if they are constantly violated? As long as one is healthy and maintaining a reasonable weight, there is really no reason to follow extreme dietary restrictions. And even if you need to follow some restrictions because of health reasons, there is no reason to deprive yourself of good, tasty food.

The best way to healthy eating is to cultivate your taste. Pay attention to the quality of the food, become a gourmet. Within reason, gourmets eat what they're in the mood for and nevertheless stay healthy. They are trim and fit enough, although they do not tend to be coat hangers. They are usually in good spirits, enjoying the finer things in life. This strengthens their immune systems and protects them from many ailments.

Instead of following prohibitions and learning to forego food, it is better to cook good balanced meals and to develop your own culinary taste. Gourmets will never succumb to unrestrained food orgies. They know that freedom has limits. But they set these limits for themselves, rather than rigidly following restrictions laid down by an "expert" who says he knows better.

Packaged recipes for the perfect lifestyle are available on every corner these days. Gourmets, however, go through the pains of working out for themselves what is good for them and what is not. They pay attention to their personal likes and dislikes, to which foods give them energy and a sense of well-being, and to which foods cause indigestion or lethargy. A diet that includes plenty of whole grains and fresh fruits and vegetables can accommodate the occasional steak or piece of chocolate cake. It's all a matter of balance. When you have paid attention to your diet for a while, an inner voice will tell you what you should eat and what you should not.

The gourmet always keeps two things in mind, the joy of eating good food and the interest in its preparation. Self-appointed nutrition apostles who preach abstinence without understanding anything about cuisine can be brushed off as mere nuisances.

Gourmets are masters of improvisation. They can prepare a feast from the remains of the weekend shopping, even on a Thursday night. Only fools assert that one needs to be wealthy to be a gourmet. Sometimes gourmets will buy expensive wines and good cuts of meat, but on other days they might create a wonderful low-cost meal out of leftovers, seasoned artfully with a lime, a little cream, sherry, and some thyme.

The Ginger Family in the Gourmet's Kitchen

Those who have been to an Arab bazaar or an Asian market know the unique aroma in the air there, and how beautiful all the spices look. Oh, this is what cinnamon, a clove, cardamom, or turmeric looks like, thinks the traveler who up to this point has seen only ground spices.

For most spices, the following applies—as soon as they are ground up and exposed to oxygen, they begin to lose their aroma and strength. Those who have ever smelled the wonderful scent of fresh homeground spices will never want to return to preground, even if grinding them does take a little extra time.

CARDAMOM

Cardamom seedpods are always sold dried. If the capsule is harvested early, it will remain tightly shut for a long time and keep the seeds inside fresh. Good quality cardamom can be recognized by the fact that the capsule is green and hard to crack. The seeds inside should be slightly sticky, very dark brown on the outside, and white on the inside. They have an intense and unique aroma.

There are cardamom plantations throughout the tropical belt, from Asia to Latin America. The principal cultivating country, however, is India. Cardamom powder should not be used in the kitchen, it is about as tasty as wood shavings. Even if it is offered in vacuum-sealed packaging, as soon as the package is opened the aroma fades and the powder becomes worthless. When cooking with cardamom, add it only toward the end of the cooking time to protect its tender aroma.

TURMERIC

Turmeric is usually offered for sale and used as a powder. It is one of the few spices that can be bought already ground without any loss in quality. The fresh bulb is not used in the kitchen. It's better that way too, since it has a strong color and will leave yellow stains on everything it touches. While the stains can be removed with oil or alcohol, the fresh bulb has no significant culinary advantage over the powder.

Ground turmeric will stain as well, but one has to work with it less and can thus reduce the risk.

Turmeric is contained in most curry mixtures, but it can be used alone. It has a good taste, although it becomes bitter after prolonged cooking. That is why turmeric or curry should be added only during the last minutes of cooking.

HOW TO WORK WITH WHOLE SPICES

Those who buy only whole spices need an electric or hand-operated spice mill. The amounts given in the recipes should be ground just before cooking. Unground spices will last for several years without losing their flavor. Volatile oils and spicy constituents remain carefully enclosed in the plant cells. Only when the cells are disrupted by mechanical means do these substances escape and dissolve in the air. Sometimes spices are roasted slightly before use. The whole spices should be dry-roasted very carefully, until they emit their scent. Place the spices in a heavy-bottomed pan over low to medium heat and stir frequently while roasting. They must not become too hot, as this will cause them to lose their aroma. After roasting, they should be allowed to cool off before being ground.

GALANGAL

Galangal is not very common outside of Southeast Asia and China. As with ginger, the whole bulb is sold, but only in Asian food stores. Most commonly you will find the big galangal there, which is white or yellow inside. While the small galangal looks the same from outside, it is a light pink inside.

Both types of galangal are found in Indonesian and Thai curries and soups. Because galangal is harder to work with and not found as readily, it is used much less often than ginger. Galangal is not suited for raw consumption as it is hard to grind and has a very strong taste.

GINGER

Both dried and fresh ginger bulbs are sold commonly. For dried ginger bulbs there are no special things to pay attention to. They are always peeled and bleached from the sun. Shortly before use you can scrape off the desired amount of ginger with a nutmeg grater. Dried ginger has a different taste from fresh ginger, sharper and more bitter. It has the character of a spice.

Ground ginger should not be bought. After the initial opening it loses its aroma rapidly. Only in the undamaged plant cells of a ginger bulb do the valuable volatile oils remain intact.

Fresh ginger has a milder taste than dried ginger. It should be juicy and free of fibers, the skin smooth and light brown, with a dull luster. How spicy ginger is and how many fibers it has is not related to the country of origin but, rather, to the point in its growth at which it was harvested. The later the harvest, the spicier the root. Early harvest results in a firm, mild, juicy bulb. If fresh ginger is added to food only shortly before serving it is unnoticeable, because it cannot develop its spice. Generally, for both ginger and galangal, the longer they cook, the spicier the food will become.

Storage of Fresh Roots Is Easy

It is always good to have fresh ginger or galangal on hand at home, and their storage presents no problems. Usually one buys more than is needed for a single meal. If an especially juicy and solid plant is offered, one should buy it to have a small reserve. Fresh bulbs last for about three weeks in the fridge. If they are wrapped in foil or plastic they will soon start to mold, but if they are left unwrapped they will soon dry out.

The best way to store fresh roots is to freeze the bulbs unpeeled. They can be used at any time; you don't even have to wait for them to thaw. Frozen ginger is easier to grate than fresh ginger, and it can be divided and peeled easily as well. Galangal, too, is much easier to handle when frozen.

Peeled, whole pieces of ginger or galangal can be marinated in Madeira, sherry, or brandy and will keep in the refrigerator for several months. The alcohol releases the spicy constituents and takes on the taste of the ginger. At the same time, the ginger also soaks up the flavor of the alcohol. This creates two modified spices that should make the gourmet happy.

According to the recipe, fresh ginger can be carefully cut with a knife, ground up, or grated. Small hand-held grinders that are easy to clean are preferable to more complicated machinery. Galangal is often merely divided into several chunks, then cooked with the food for a longer period of time. Before serving it should be picked out of the dish so as not to put the guest in the awkward position of trying to eat the hard pieces.

Hot, Sweet, and Rich

Most dishes that are prepared with the ginger family are spicy, especially if the recipes contain chili as well. This spiciness needs a counterpoint that complements and restrains it. This counterpoint can be anything sweet. It ensures harmony in the pot, as can be observed with almost all Asian dishes. Be it Thai, Indian, Indonesian, Vietnamese, or Chinese, sweetness plays a large complementary role. In addition to the known combination of sweet and sour, the taste pair sweet and spicy appears in many exotic dishes as well.

Sugar, honey, raisins, sweet chutneys, and almond flour are the most important sweetening substances.

Of course, other sweeteners can also be used. In Thai cuisine, palm sugar is preferred, since it not only is sweet but also has its own aroma.

Depending on the sweetening ingredient used, the character of the sweetness will change. Sugar and honey spread evenly throughout the dish, whereas raisins retain their sweetness until they are chewed. The almond flour eases the spiciness in two ways; besides being sweet, it also contains fat.

Fat neutralizes the spicy constituents, while water does not. That is why not even a cool beer will relieve the fire they cause in the throat. One spoonful of yogurt, however, will extinguish it immediately, since yogurt contains fat. Yogurt, coconut cream, almond flour, butter, and butter fat thus all contribute to a balanced curry dish as much as the sweet ingredients do.

All Asian dishes are based on the proper balance between spiciness, sweetness, and fat. The most common spices, aside from ginger, turmeric, cardamom, and galangal, are cloves, cumin, mustard seeds, fenugreek, star anise, fennel, coriander, and cinnamon.

More Taste, Less Salt

Salt can easily be avoided in most Asian recipes—as opposed to German, Italian, or French cuisines, which rely heavily on salt and pepper. Many European dishes taste boring and empty if they contain too little salt.

Anyone who has had to switch to a low-sodium diet for health reasons can attest to this.

In Asian dishes, however, even a normal amount of salt can disrupt the delicate balance between the ingredients. Spicy dishes should thus be salted only lightly, and even then only with care.

Asian dishes, with their plethora of spices, are a surprise for all those that have to forego salt for health reasons. Even people who should reduce the consumption of fried foods are cared for, as in many Asian recipes the meat is only steamed or boiled.

It is a prejudice that spices are hard to digest! On the contrary, they are healthy and stimulate the digestion. This is especially true for the members of the ginger family. Thus they prove that good medicine does not have to taste bad.

Vegetarians also love spices. It is an accomplishment of Indian cuisine to have created truly tasty vegetarian dishes. They would not be possible without ginger, turmeric, and cardamom.

Those who have tried these spices once will soon start to experiment and compose their own favorite recipes. This book only provides a few suggestions, the rest is left to the improvisation of our readers.

5
The Recipes

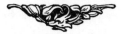

Drinks First

Healthy cooking with the ginger family starts with
some recipes for coffee, tea, and an aperitif. Hot drinks
and soups made with ginger, galangal, and cardamom
not only taste great but also release the healing and
stimulating effects of these spices. And a ginger vinegar as an aperitif is the ideal companion for an opu-
lent feast.

COFFEE ORIENTAL

Cardamom is a traditional coffee spice. Those who
want to know how it would taste by itself should spice
one pot of coffee with crushed cardamom seeds. Even
diluted coffee becomes a delicacy with cardamom.
This is of interest for all those who do not enjoy strong
coffee. Arabs drink a lot of coffee and thus have been
spicing it with cardamom for centuries. That is why a
large part of the worldwide cardamom harvest is consumed by Arabs.

Everyone has seen a typical Arab coffeepot before: a balloon-shaped container made out of brass or aluminum with a slender neck and a very thin spout. In Arab recipes the cardamom seeds are placed in the spout, where the coffee flows past them during pouring.

Coffee with Cardamom

1. Use 1 cardamom seedpod per cup of coffee. Open the capsule, peel the seeds out of their shell, and crush them slightly.
2. Place the seeds in the coffeepot.
3. Prepare the coffee as usual. The seeds can remain in the pot until the coffee is finished.

Variation: Good news for all tea-drinkers—cardamom is also a good spice for black tea. Prepare as usual; simply add the crushed cardamom seeds to the teapot before adding the water.

WAKE UP WITH GINGER

Those who have low blood pressure have a hard time getting started in the mornings. Here it pays to change habits and to begin the day in a different way. People who have a hard time getting up in the mornings should drink their morning coffee in bed before getting up. Coffee in bed goes well with two or three pieces of bittersweet chocolate melted slowly on the tongue while the coffee flows over it. Spicing the coffee with some ginger also stimulates the heart and lets the blood flow more quickly. Ayurvedic medicine even says that an early breakfast can be left out entirely, since it slows down circulation unnecessarily and makes one feel tired right after getting up.

Hot Ginger-Milk Coffee

1. Prepare the coffee as usual. Heat the milk but do not boil it. Beat the milk until foamy; the foam prevents a skin from forming on top of the milk.
2. Pour milk and coffee into a cup and add honey or sweetener according to taste.
3. Scrape one dried ginger root with a nutmeg grater. Add the freshly grated ginger to the cup and stir briefly. Start with one knife tip of ginger per cup, you can increase this dosage later should you wish.

CAUGHT A COLD? NO PROBLEM.

"With medications they last seven days, without them one week," is a saying about colds. Ginger facilitates the healing and can even prevent the infection from taking hold in the first place. Thus, buy ginger as soon as you notice the first symptoms (runny nose, scratchy throat, headaches, and body aches).

Hot Ginger Tea

Makes 2 cups of tea.

2 tablespoons fresh ginger
2 cups water
$1/4$ cup milk
honey according to taste

1. Peel the ginger and grate into rough pieces. Add to the cold water and bring the mixture to a boil. Let the mixture boil for about 10 minutes.
2. Add the milk and sweeten according to taste. Bring the entire mixture to a boil again. Strain out the ginger.
3. Lie down in bed, cover up, and drink the tea as hot as possible.

A good everyday drink is a tea made from lemon verbena leaves. The plant comes from South America, it adds a pleasant lemon taste to dishes, and as a tea stimulates the kidneys and refreshes and quenches thirst. Lemon verbena and ginger go well together.

Lemon Verbena Tea with Ginger
Makes 1 quart of tea.

1 whole piece dried ginger
3 black peppercorns
3 tablespoons dried lemon verbena leaves
1 quart water
milk and honey according to taste

1. Grind the ginger and the pepper.
2. Put the lemon verbena leaves and the spices in a pan and pour the boiling water over them. Cover, keep warm, and allow to steep for 10 minutes.
3. Pour through a sieve and drink while hot. Milk and honey round off the taste nicely, but the tea also tastes good unsweetened.

GOOD OLD FRIENDS— VINEGAR AND GINGER

Vinegar was already well known six thousand years ago in ancient China, Mesopotamia, and Egypt. Today it is popular again as a healing substance. The following recipe adds new flavor to salads; it can also be drunk as an aperitif.

Ginger Vinegar
Makes 1 quart.

1 teaspoon fresh ginger

1 teaspoon sugar

1 quart white wine vinegar or sherry vinegar

1. Peel the ginger and chop fine.
2. Mix all ingredients and place in a clean non-metalic container.
3. After two weeks, pour it through a coffee filter into clean bottles.

Hot Soups for Cold Days

With a hot soup in the stomach, the world looks a much better place. It makes you full, and warmth spreads through the entire body. It is good as a small lunchtime snack, as an energy source, and as an appetizer for a larger menu. There is a recipe for every occasion. Ginger, cardamom, turmeric, and galangal do not belong in every soup, but some recipes are literally aching for the addition of one of these spices.

GINGER AND GALANGAL IN LOVE WITH A CHARMING THAI SOUP

There is only one soup in which one can adequately appreciate galangal. It comes from Thailand and is among the best that soups have to offer. The basis of this soup is a homemade chicken broth, which one should really always have in store. You can produce it in large quantities, freeze it, and then use it as a base for chicken soup, as well as for poultry and vegetable dishes.

Chicken Broth

Makes about 2 quarts of stock.

1 5-pound chicken
1-inch piece of fresh ginger
1-inch piece of fresh galangal
2 cloves garlic
3 green onions
1 stem lemongrass
1 star anise pod
2 tablespoons fish sauce
3 dried red chili peppers
2 quarts water

1. Wash the chicken inside and out and let it drip dry.
2. Peel the ginger and galangal and cut into thick slices. Peel and crush the garlic and slice the green onions.
3. Put all ingredients into a pot. Fill with cold water. Cover the pot, bring to a boil, and simmer for 3 hours.
4. Hang a sieve over a large bowl. Pour off the broth and let it cool down. The fat will rise to the surface.
5. Carefully take off the fat, place it in a jar and store it in the refrigerator. It will last a long time and is excellent for frying chicken or sautéeing vegetables.
6. Freeze the broth and thaw when needed.

Tom-Kha-Gai Soup

Serves 4.

1 pound chicken breasts

3 tablespoons cornstarch

5 mushrooms

2$^1/_2$ cups chicken broth

1 tablespoon peanut oil

1 bunch green onions

2-inch piece of fresh galangal

2 tablespoons ground ginger

2 stems lemongrass

3 tablespoons fish sauce*

3 tablespoons lemon juice

1$^2/_3$ cup coconut cream

salt to taste

freshly ground black pepper

fresh Thai basil

1. Wash the chicken breasts and dry them.
   Remove tendons and fat. Cut across the grain
   into bite-sized strips. Dredge in cornstarch and
   set aside.
2. Wash the mushrooms. If they are older, remove
   the top skin. Cut into thin slices.

---

*Fish sauce is an Indonesian condiment found in Asian
specialty markets.

3. Cut the green onions into fine slices and sauté briefly in oil in the soup pot. Add the chicken broth and heat.

4. Peel the galangal and cut into thin slices. Peel the ginger and grate fine. Cut the lemongrass into very thin rings. Put everything in the pot and add the fish sauce.

5. Briefly bring to a boil. Remove from heat and let sit for 10 minutes, then mix in the coconut cream. Return to a boil and cook on medium heat.

6. Season the mushrooms and the chicken with salt and freshly ground pepper, and add to the soup. Let everything boil for about 5 minutes. In order to keep the meat and the mushrooms tender, do not boil longer.

7. Wash and dry the basil and cut it into strips. Add to the soup before serving and let it sit for 5 minutes without cooking.

Tip: Coconut cream is available unsweetened in cans or as instant powder. Both forms are delicious and aromatic, and they are practical to use, as the preparation of coconut cream from fresh coconut is difficult, expensive, and sometimes—due to a lack of nuts—not even possible. Grated coconut is no replacement for coconut cream.

PUMPKIN FOREVER

Pumpkin is an American vegetable. It was domesticated about fifty-five hundred years ago in Latin America, Peru, and on the east coast of North America. The meat of pumpkin shines in various shades of orange and yellow. It is excellent for the preparation of visually appealing soups. You do not need turmeric to enhance the color, but ginger is necessary for flavor.

Pumpkin Cream Soup with Apple and Ginger
Serves 4.

1 medium-sized pumpkin

3 tablespoons butter

1 cup water

1 apple

2 tablespoons fresh ginger

1 teaspoon freshly ground black pepper

1 teaspoon salt

2 tablespoons sugar

2 tablespoons calvados*

1. Peel the pumpkin, remove the seeds, and cut into slices.
2. Place butter, water, and pumpkin in a pot, cover it, and allow it to cook.

---

*Calvados is an apple jack made in Calvados, France.

3. Peel the apple, remove the core, and cut it into quarters. Peel the ginger and grate it fine.
4. When the pumpkin starts to soften, add all the seasonings and continue cooking for another 15 minutes.
5. Puree everything in a blender and add the calvados. Add salt and pepper according to taste.

Variation: Every year there comes asparagus season. After cooking the asparagus in lightly salted water with a bit of butter added in, do not pour the water out, but rather keep it. Divide it into small containers and put them in the freezer. The water saved from one asparagus dinner doubles as a great soup stock and will last for a long time. This stock goes well with the soup mentioned above. You can substitute the asparagus stock for the water and the calvados.

Born for Each Other— Meat and Ginger

Meat and ginger are a combination that has been appreciated for millennia. This is true not only from a culinary point of view, but from a medical point of view as well. Because meat goes bad quickly it is, and always has been, a health risk. Ginger diminishes the effects of food poisoning, which is significant in developing countries where not every household has a refrigerator. Ginger has a place in modern cuisine too because it also tenderizes meat.

Lamb with Spinach, Ginger, and Cardamom
Serves 4 to 6.

2 pounds lean lamb
2 teaspoons fresh ginger
2 cloves garlic
1 pound spinach, chopped (frozen is fine)
4 tablespoons butter ($^1/_2$ stick)
2 teaspoons curry powder (see chart at end of
this section)
2 cardamom seeds
1 cinnamon stick
$^1/_2$ teaspoon cayenne pepper
$^1/_2$ cup plain yogurt
1 tablespoon almonds
$^1/_2$ teaspoon nutmeg
3 tablespoons cream

The Recipes

1. Wash the lamb, dry it, and cut it into bite-sized pieces.
2. Peel the ginger and grate or chop fine. Peel and crush the garlic. Mix both with the lamb. Let sit for 20 minutes.
3. Put the meat with the marinade into a pot. Add cold water until it is completely covered. Bring to a boil and simmer for about 30 minutes.
4. In the meantime, thaw the spinach in another pot and steam it for a few minutes. If the spinach is only roughly chopped, it should be pureed in a blender.
5. Take the meat out of the pot, drain it in a colander, and save the marinade. Place the meat on kitchen towels, dry it off well, and briefly suaté it in the fat.
6. Add all spices except for the nutmeg and almonds. Cook the meat with the yogurt for about 8 minutes until it has completely absorbed the yogurt and there is barely any liquid left in the pot.
7. Add spinach, almonds, nutmeg, and about 1 cup of the marinade. Let it simmer for about 8 minutes while keeping the lid tightly shut. Mix in the cream and carefully heat it again.
8. Serve with basmati rice.

HOW TO MAKE YOUR OWN CURRY POWDER

The word *curry* or *kari* comes from southern India and literally translates into "sauce." Today "curry" is an umbrella term for all opulently spiced Far Eastern dishes. Curry is also the name of a mixture of spices that is available in every grocery store. However, it is composed mainly of turmeric, so there is a lot missing in terms of taste.

Ready-made spices are hardly used at all in India. Indian cooks use a different mixture of spices for every curry dish and prepare this mixture only shortly before cooking. Of course, you can prepare your own stock of spice mix and use it up as you go along. However, the older the powder gets, the more flavor it will lose. It should not be used for longer than two or three weeks.

All of the ingredients, with the exception of the turmeric, are roasted in a pan without fat. They must not get too hot or they will burn. As soon as the spices start to release their aroma they should be removed from the heat, allowed to cool off a bit, and then all finely ground together in a spice mill. Turmeric powder is added only after this.

With the help of the chart at the end of this section various types of curry can be prepared. As a beginner you can experiment with all the variations. Over time you will learn which mixture goes best with which dish, but there are no set rules for these correspondences. The curry variations listed in the chart are merely suggestions and are not limiting. Those who like to improvise will enjoy the preparation and use of various curry powders.

Recipes that call for "garam masala" or "Madras curry" fulfill the desire for simple, quick solutions. They are not acceptable to curry connoisseurs since they reduce a wonderful authentic combination to something that does not actually exist anymore. That is because the more recipes you read, the more combinations you will find for "garam masala" or "Madras curry." Many cookbook authors do not even list the contents of the combination anymore, as they expect that you will buy the ready-made mixture.

With the following curry tables you can prepare eleven different curry mixtures. The numbers in the top row number the combinations, the other numbers indicate the weight proportions.

CURRY TABLE I

Ingredients Mixture	Weight Proportions				
	1	2	3	4	5
Black pepper	1	1	1	1	2
Chili	1	2	1	1	3
Cloves	1	1	0	0	0
Cinnamon	0	2	0	0	0
Cardamom	1	1	0	0	0
Coriander	8	6	8	8	8
Cumin	0	2	2	0	1
Fenugreek	0	1	2	0	1
Ginger	1	0	1	2	0
Nutmeg	0	1	0	0	0
Mustard seeds	0	0	1	0	0
Poppy seeds	0	0	1	0	0
Turmeric	9	0	5	9	4

CURRY TABLE II

Ingredients Mixture	Weight Proportions					
	1	2	3	4	5	6
Black pepper	2	1	1	1	8	4
Chili	2	6	8	4	0	0
Cloves	0	0	0	1	2	2
Cinnamon	0	0	1	1	2	2
Cardamom	0	0	1	1	2	4
Coriander	8	8	8	8	8	8
Cumin	1	1	4	2	6	4
Fenugreek	0	2	0	1	0	0
Ginger	1	0	0	0	0	0
Nutmeg	0	0	0	0	0	0
Mustard seeds	2	0	0	0	0	0
Poppy seeds	0	0	0	0	0	0
Turmeric	2	2	3	3	0	0

Friends of Asian cuisine love poultry. It is the ideal ingredient for refined creations and remains tender and juicy when it is placed in a sauce or soup only shortly before being served. This simple and mild preparation is also very healthy, as the chicken is not fried in fat.

Chicken in Coconut Sauce with Broccoli
Serves 4.

1 bunch broccoli

1³/₄ cup coconut cream

1 teaspoon palm sugar

1 teaspoon salt

1 tablespoon fish sauce

1 tablespoon lemon juice

1 tablespoon freshly ground ginger

2 tablespoons curry powder #10 (see previous chart)

¹/₂ pound chicken breast

2 teaspoons cornstarch

1 bunch Thai basil

1. Let the broccoli, sugar, salt, fish sauce, lemon juice, and spices simmer in the coconut cream until the vegetables are soft.

2. Cut the meat across the grain into bite-sized strips, dredge with cornstarch, add salt and pepper. Add to the sauce and allow to simmer on low heat for 5 minutes.

3. Wash the basil and cut it lengthwise into strips. Mix in shortly before serving, do not boil.

4. Best served with basmati rice.

Chutneys—Sweets to Complement Meats

The following pineapple chutney and the pumpkin-apple-carrot chutney go well with cold pork or chicken, as well as with boiled ham. After the jars are sealed they should be set aside for one month in a dark, cool, dry place to let the flavors "marry." After opening the chutneys will last for about one year if refrigerated.

Pineapple Chutney

Makes about 3 cups.

1 cinnamon stick

2 teaspoons cardamom seeds

$^1/_2$ teaspoon whole black peppercorns

4 cloves

1 whole ripe pineapple

$^1/_2$ cup ginger vinegar (refer to earlier recipe)

1 teaspoon fresh ginger

1 cup sugar

1. Roast the spices in a pan until they begin to release their aroma. Allow them to cool off a bit and then grind fine.
2. Peel the pineapple, removing the eyes and the core. Chop up the pineapple meat and collect the juice that is released.
3. Heat the juice with the vinegar, the spices, and the ginger and let it simmer for 5 minutes.

4. Add the pineapple pieces and let them simmer until they are completely soft.
5. Mix in the sugar. Raise the heat as soon as it is dissolved. Cook for about 30 minutes, until the mixture has thickened.
6. Pour into hot, sterilized canning jars and seal with acid-resistant lids.

Pumpkin-Apple-Carrot Chutney
Makes about 4 cups.

1/2 pound pumpkin
2 medium apples
2 medium carrots
1 onion
1 tablespoon fresh ginger
1 teaspoon cumin
3 teaspoons coriander
2 teaspoons cardamom seeds
1/2 teaspoon whole black peppercorns
1 teaspoon turmeric powder
2 teaspoons salt
1 1/3 cups sugar
2/3 cup raisins
1 1/4 cups apple cider vinegar
2 tablespoons calvados*

1. Peel the apples and the pumpkin, remove the seeds, and chop into small pieces. Peel the

---

*Calvados is an apple jack made in Calvados, France.

carrots and cut into long thin strips. Slice the onion into thin rings. Peel the ginger and grate fine.

2. Dry roast the cumin, coriander, cardamom, and pepper in a pan without fat, until they start to release their aroma. Let them cool off a bit and then grind fine together. Add the turmeric powder.

3. Carefully heat all ingredients in vinegar and calvados while stirring, continue until the sugar has dissolved. Cook for about 30 minutes until the mixture thickens.

4. Pour into hot, sterilized canning jars and seal with acid-resistant lids. Store for two months in a cool, dark, dry place before opening.

Ginger and Fish

For a long time it was considered a culinary faux pas to spice fish with ginger. It was believed that the delicate aroma of the fish would be dominated by the strong flavor of ginger. This belief ends the first time you eat a fish curry. When fish is spiced with ginger or used in a curry dish, moderately priced fish—perch for example—will suffice.

Perch with Ginger and Coconut
Serves 4.

1 1/2 pounds perch
6 teaspoons lemon juice
1 teaspoon cumin
1/2 teaspoon fennel seeds
3 tablespoons grated coconut
1 teaspoon fresh ginger
2 cloves garlic
1 onion
1 teaspoon turmeric
2 tablespoons butter
1 3/4 cups water
2 tablespoons chopped cilantro (fresh green
coriander leaves)

1. Wash the fillets and cut into slices 1 inch thick. Drizzle with half of the lemon juice and set aside.
2. Roast the cumin, fennel, and grated coconut in a pan without fat until they start to release

their aroma. Let them cool off a bit and grind
into a powder.

3. Peel the ginger, garlic, and onion, puree
   together in a blender, then add the spices,
   turmeric, and the remaining lemon juice.
4. Fry this paste in butter while stirring; add water
   and bring to a boil; let cook for 6 minutes.
5. Add the fish and half of the cilantro. Cook on
   low heat for 6 minutes, until the fish is done. Do
   not stir or the fish will fall apart.
6. Decorate with the remaining coriander. Serve
   with basmati rice.

Tonka-Ginger Perch
Serves 4.

1 1/2 pounds perch
salt
freshly ground black pepper
3 carrots
2 teaspoons fresh ginger
1 onion
1 clove garlic
1 tablespoon vegetable oil
1/2 cup water
1 1/2 cups white wine
1/2 cup fish stock
3/4 cup cream

$^1/_3$ tonka bean (see box on page 107)
2 tablespoons fresh basil
1 tablespoon fresh cilantro (coriander leaves)

1. Wash the fish, pat it dry. Rub with salt and freshly ground pepper and set aside.
2. Peel and slice the carrots. Peel and chop the ginger, onion, and garlic..
3. Slightly steam carrots, ginger, and onion, add the garlic at the end. Deglaze the pan with water, white wine, and stock. Bring to a boil and simmer for 15 minutes.
4. Increase the heat and boil to reduce to half the volume of liquid. Add cream.
5. Continue to boil until the mixture thickens. Add the tonka bean using a nutmeg grater. Add salt and freshly ground pepper to taste.
6. Arrange vegetables into a bed on the bottom of the pot and place the fish on top of them. Cover and simmer for 10 minutes on low heat.
7. Wash and chop the basil and cilantro.
8. Place the fillets on preheated plates. Add the basil and cilantro to the sauce and remove from heat.
9. Serve with noodles or basmati rice.

Tonka-Ginger Shrimp
Serves 4.

2 pounds shrimp

1 celeriac root

3 carrots

1 onion

2 leeks, white part only

1 small bunch parsley

1-inch piece fresh ginger

1 clove garlic

1 tablespoon vegetable oil

6 twigs fresh thyme

2 twigs fresh rosemary

10 black peppercorns, ground

1 bay leaf

2 cups white wine

1 cup water

$^3/_4$ cup cream

about $^1/_3$ tonka bean (see box on page 107)

1. Peel and devein the shrimp, wash them, and pat dry. Set aside.
2. Peel and chop the celeriac, carrots, onion, garlic, and ginger. Trim and chop the leeks and parsley.
3. Briefly roast the shrimp shells on high heat, add the vegetables and start to steam the mixture. Now add the spices, the ground peppercorns, and the bay leaf.
4. Deglaze the pan with wine, add water. Bring to

a brief boil and then simmer for 30 minutes on medium heat.

5. Strain the stock into a different pot. Reduce by half at high heat.
6. Add cream, continue reducing the sauce until it turns slightly grainy.
7. Grate the tonka bean directly into the sauce and boil for 5 more minutes.
8. Add salt and pepper according to taste.
9. Add the peeled shrimp to the sauce. Simmer on medium heat for about 3 minutes until the shrimp turn red-orange. Do not boil them or they will become tough.
10. Serve with noodles and a dry white wine.

TONKA BEANS ARE SOUTH AMERICAN

The tonka bean tree *(Dipteryx odorata)* grows in Venezuela, Guyana, and Brazil. Hard-shelled, plum-like seedpods will develop out of its aromatic flowers. The fruit is opened, the beans are removed and dried in the sun. These beans contain the fragrant compound coumarin. After drying they are marinated in rum for twenty-four hours, which causes them to swell and turn black. They are dried a second time, which causes them to shrivel up again. They are now covered with white coumarin crystals, which are responsible for their unique aroma. Tonka bean goes well with white meat, fish, and shellfish.

Eat More Vegetables!

Many people would eat more vegetables if they enjoyed them more. Vegetables are often badly prepared, either half raw or overcooked, too salty or too bland. Many years ago now, a long-forgotten French chef pronounced that, in order to preserve their own flavors, vegetables should not be seasoned. Cabbage should taste like cabbage, potatoes like potatoes, period. This is ridiculous. Cabbage especially enjoys company in the pot. And leeks, sweet potatoes, and pumpkins welcome visits from the ginger family.

Savoy Cabbage with Ginger and Cardamom
Serves 2.

1 savoy cabbage

1 tablespoon butter

1 cup vegetable broth

1 cup water

1 star anise pod

1 tablespoon fresh ginger

1 teaspoon cardamom seeds

1 teaspoon ground black pepper

$1/_2$ cup cream

1 pinch nutmeg (grated)

1 pinch salt

1. Remove the outer savoy cabbage leaves, halve the cabbage, and cut out the core. Cut the rest into $1/_4$-inch strips.

2. Sauté cabbage in the butter.
3. Pour the vegetable broth over the cabbage.
   Add the star anise whole, stir, and close the lid.
   Let simmer for about 30 minutes.
4. Peel the ginger and grate fine. Remove the
   cardamom seeds from the pod and crush them.
5. Add the vegetables and the cream to the savoy
   cabbage and simmer for another 10 minutes.
6. Add salt and nutmeg according to taste.
7. Serve with boiled potatoes, mashed potatoes,
   or rice.

A Thai Vegetable Mix
Serves 4.

1 pound yellow pumpkin

$1/_3$ pound red garnet yams

$1/_3$ pound green beans

$1/_3$ pound green cabbage

1 small onion

2 cloves garlic

3 tablespoons sunflower oil

$1/_4$ pound tomatoes

1 red chili pepper

$1/_4$ of a wild lime*

*Both the fruit and the leaves of the Far Eastern wild lime tree *(Citrus hystrix)* are common ingredients in Thai cuisine. They can be obtained from Asian specialty food markets, where the Thai word for the leaves is *bai makrut* and the word for citrus products in general is *djeruk purut.*

3 wild lime leaves
3 teaspoons palm sugar
1 teaspoon salt
1 tablespoon fish sauce
1 cup coconut cream
1 cup chicken broth (see recipe on page 89)
2 teaspoons lemon juice

1. Peel the pumpkin and remove the seeds.
   Peel yams and cut both into bite-sized cubes.
2. Wash the beans, trim the ends, and halve
   them. Cut the cabbage into $1/4$-inch strips.
3. Peel and chop the onion. Sauté in the oil until
   transparent. Peel and mince the garlic and
   sauté briefly.
4. Add the remaining ingredients and simmer for
   about 5 minutes.
5. Add the cabbage and beans and simmer for
   another 10 minutes. Now add the rest of the
   vegetables, stir well, and simmer until done.
6. Serve with basmati rice.

The Recipes

No other vegetable is as open to exotic treatment as leeks are. In perfect harmony, ginger and leeks perform a culinary duet.

A Duet for Ginger and Leeks
Serves 2.

4 large leeks
1 cup vegetable broth
2 tablespoons fresh ginger
$^1/_2$ teaspoon black peppercorns, cracked
1 pinch salt
$^1/_2$ cup cream

1. Peel the leeks, halve them lengthwise, wash well, and cut it into small pieces.
2. Simmer the leeks in the vegetable broth until tender.
3. Peel the ginger and grate fine. Add to the leeks with the cracked pepper.
4. Mix in the cream and add salt to taste. Cook a few more minutes until the sauce thickens.
5. Serve with basmati rice.

SWEET AND CRISPY

A culinary excursion to the Caribbean provides an interesting change for vegetable lovers, as everything is prepared differently. This dish can be served as an appetizer or as a main course.

Pineapple Sweet-Potato Gratin
Serves 4.

5 large sweet potatoes
1 2-cup can pineapple
$1/2$ teaspoon nutmeg (grated)
2 tablespoons fresh ginger
2 teaspoons cinnamon
3 tablespoons dark rum

1. Cook the potatoes "al dente," peel, and slice them.
2. Drain the pineapple, then break it into small pieces.
3. Grate the nutmeg, peel and grate the ginger.
4. Mix the pineapple with all the spices and the rum, place on top of the potatoes.
5. Preheat the oven to 350ºF and bake for 15 minutes.

GINGER FOR KIDS

Spicy food is often not appropriate for the tender taste buds of children. Thus, many Asian recipes have to be "de-spiced" or toned down when served to children. They will tolerate only a limited amount of spice. With the following gratin you can discreetly test the ginger tolerance of your children.

Semolina Casserole with Raisins
Serves 4.

1 quart milk
1 cup semolina
1 pinch salt
1 pound ricotta cheese
4–5 eggs
1 teaspoon grated lemon peel
1 tablespoon freshly ground ginger
1 cup raisins
$^3/_4$ cup sugar
$^2/_3$ cup chopped almonds
bread crumbs
2 tablespoons butter

1. Heat the milk. Add semolina and salt and cook while stirring until you have a stiff paste. Set aside and allow to cool.
2. Preheat the oven to 350°F. Separate the eggs. Beat the egg whites until soft peaks form and set aside.

3. Mix the ricotta with the egg yolks, lemon peel, ginger, raisins, sugar, and almonds. Add the semolina and finally fold in the beaten egg whites.
4. Turn out into a buttered casserole dish. Sprinkle with bread crumbs and the remaining butter. Bake for about 1 hour.

Variation: Instead of raisins, you can also peel 2 apples, remove their seeds, and divide each into 8 pieces. The pieces are dispersed in the mass evenly and baked.

AFTERNOON SNACKS

In the middle of the afternoon, regardless of whether you are in the office or at home, you have less energy and would appreciate a nap. But most of us have to tough it out somehow. The body yearns for food. You hear its message clearly—give me something sweet and I'll be happy again.

Fruits and raw vegetables do not satisfy the hunger, as they are no replacement for candy. Those who want to avoid reaching for chocolate but still want to satisfy this hunger should try sweetened ginger carrots sautéed in butter. You can prepare a stash the night before and eat as much as you want the next day.

Sweet Ginger Carrots

4 large carrots
1 teaspoon fresh ginger
3 tablespoons butter
2 teaspoons sugar
freshly ground black pepper
salt

1. Peel the carrots. Peel the ginger and grate fine.
2. Heat butter in a pan, mix in the ginger and the whole carrots. Stir, cover, and sauté on low heat for 10 minutes.
3. Add the sugar, freshly ground pepper, and salt to taste. Stir and sauté for another 10 minutes.
4. Put the carrots with the sauce in a covered container and keep cold. It is fine if the carrots are still crisp inside. Add some vinegar before eating, if you like.

Mango Apple Salad

Serves 2.

1 mango
2 apples
2 tablespoons lemon juice
1 tablespoon fresh ginger
$^1/_4$ cup olive oil
$^1/_4$ cup apple cider vinegar
1 teaspoon mustard
1 teaspoon cardamom seeds
$^1/_2$ teaspoon sugar
$^1/_2$ teaspoon salt
1 pinch black pepper

1. Peel the mango and the apples, then dice them. Drizzle with half the lemon juice, and refrigerate.
2. Peel the ginger and grind it into a fine paste. Take the cardamom seeds out of their pod, grind them fine or crush them.
3. Mix ginger, oil, vinegar, the remaining lemon juice, mustard, cardamom, sugar, salt, and pepper.
4. Spread over the chilled fruits, mix thoroughly, and allow to settle for $^1/_2$ hour.

WHAT TO COOK WHEN
THE CUPBOARD IS BARE

Sometimes you feel hungry, but the fridge is empty. It's raining and you don't want to go outside. On days like these it pays to have the staple ingredients for the following recipe on hand.

Dal Baht—Red Lentils with Basmati Rice
Serves 4.

$^3/_4$ cup red lentils

2 potatoes

2 carrots

1 clove garlic

2 teaspoons fresh ginger

1 vegetable bouillon cube

2 teaspoons cumin

1 teaspoon cardamom seeds

2 teaspoons ground turmeric

1 dried chili

2 teaspoons honey

1 bay leaf

$^1/_3$ cup raisins

1 tablespoon vegetable oil

4 cups water

1. Clean the lentils, looking carefully for stones. Briefly wash them in cold water and set them aside.
2. Peel and chop the potatoes and carrots. Peel

and chop garlic and ginger. Heat the water and dissolve the bouillon cube in 1 cup of it.

3. Grind the cumin and cardamom seeds in a spice mill and mix them with the turmeric powder.

4. Heat the oil. Gently break up the chili and sauté with the ginger, then add the garlic and carrots.

5. Add the broth, bay leaf, and raisins, as well as 2 cups of the warm water. Stir well and simmer on low heat for 5 minutes.

6. Add lentils, spices, and potatoes. Add the remaining water. The lentils will absorb it entirely over time.

7. If the mixture becomes too stiff, add more water.

8. Cook until the lentils are soft.

9. Serve with plain yogurt and basmati rice.

Hint: When legumes (with the exception of lentils or split peas) are soaked the day before, and then cooked in fresh water after discarding the soaking water, they will not cause flatulence and can thus be eaten even by people who have trouble digesting legumes. Lentils and split peas are faster cooking than other legumes and don't require soaking. Ginger also helps to control flatulence.

BASMATI RICE

In Asia rice is a staple food and the cuisine of this region could not be imagined without it. From Peking to Surabaya, from Manila to Karachi, the water-loving grain is the staple food. The star among Asian types of rice is basmati. No other rice smells or tastes as good, but no other is as particular to prepare either.

Basmati is prepared differently than is the American parboiled rice, or the longer Patna rice from India. Basmati rice must not boil for very long, it expands quickly in salted cooking water and absorbs it completely. This ensures its staying fluffy and prevents stickiness. It is thus important to use the proper amount of water. Basmati should always be washed before cooking.

How to Cook Basmati Rice

1. Wash the rice and let it drain in a colander. Place in cold water. Use $^3/_4$ cup water for $^1/_2$ cup rice for one portion.
2. Add salt and cover. Bring to a boil and let boil for about 1 minute. Then take the pot off the stove, keep it warm, and allow the rice to sit.
3. If the pot is well insulated, the rice will be ready after 20 minutes without any additional heat. If the time is up and the rice is not ready yet, place the pot on a flame at low heat until all the water evaporates and the the rice is fluffy.

Basmati and the Spice Lilies

Ginger and galangal: Cook a few pieces of peeled ginger or galangal together with the rice. This increases the aroma of the rice while the ginger or galangal taste remains in the background. Remove the pieces before serving.

Turmeric: If you add 1 teaspoon turmeric to the water, it will turn the rice yellow without changing the taste.

Cardamom: In India, entire cardamom pods are often added to the water. They too are removed before eating but contribute to the aroma of the rice.

Cookies, Cakes, and Crèmes

Ginger and cardamom are spices that can be used for almost any dessert. They are a good counterpoint to the sugar, because the spice lilies will clean what it clogs. They also help with the digestion of the preceding meal.

Ginger Coconut Mounds
Makes about 3 dozen cookies.

1 teaspoon fresh ginger

1 cup grated coconut

1 vanilla bean

$1^1/_2$ cups butter

$1^1/_2$ cups sugar

2 eggs

1 tablespoon rum

1 teaspoon baking powder

$4^1/_2$ cups flour

1. Peel the ginger and grate fine. Cut the vanilla bean lengthwise and scrape out the seeds.
2. Add vanilla seeds, ginger, and coconut to butter and beat until it is fluffy.
3. Mix the baking powder and the flour and add to mixture.
4. Place dough in a pastry bag and squeeze out mounds onto a greased baking sheet. If the dough is too thick, add some rum.
5. Bake in a preheated 350°F oven for about 15 minutes.

Orange Curd Cake

Serves 4.

1 organic orange

3 eggs

1 teaspoon fresh ginger

1 cardamom seedpod

1 vanilla bean

$^1/_2$ cup milk

$^1/_3$ cup plain yogurt

$1^1/_3$ cups sugar

$^1/_3$ cup flour

1. Wash the orange and grate the zest.
2. Separate the eggs. Beat the yolks until foamy.
3. Peel the ginger and grate fine, open the cardamom pod and crush the seeds fine. Cut open the vanilla bean lengthwise and scrape out the seeds.
4. Mix all of the ingredients above with the yogurt and milk. Then add 1 cup of sugar and the flour. Beat until smooth.
5. Beat the egg whites stiff with the remaining sugar and fold in carefully.
6. Turn into a buttered bundt pan and bake for about 30 minutes in a preheated 350ºF oven. The cake is ready when it has a nice golden brown color.

Date Cookies

Makes about 30 cookies.

For the filling:

1³/₄ cups candied dates
1 tablespoon fresh ginger
1 cup water

For the dough:

1 teaspoon cardamom seeds
1 cup (2 sticks) butter
3¹/₂ cups flour
1 tablespoon rose water
2 tablespoons milk
powdered sugar
chopped pistachio nuts

1. Chop the dates, peel the ginger and grate fine. Then add water and heat while stirring until the mixture thickens.
2. Open the cardamom pod, take out the seeds and crush them.
3. Cut the butter into the flour. Add the rose water, cardamom, and milk. Knead the dough until it is soft and smooth. Let it sit in the refrigerator for 20 minutes.
4. Form about thirty balls, flatten them slightly and make a dent in the middle. Put a little of the date mixture in each indentation and close the dough over it, forming oval cookies.
5. Bake in the oven at 325°F for about 30 minutes.
6. Sprinkle with powdered sugar and pistachios.

Orange Curd Crème

Serves 4.

2 organic oranges
$^1/_2$ cup sugar
1 cardamom seedpod
1 teaspoon fresh ginger
3 sheets white gelatin*
$1^1/_4$ ounces marzipan
$^3/_4$ cup yogurt
$^1/_2$ cup heavy cream

1. Grate the zest of the oranges, then squeeze out the orange juice. Boil the juice together with the zest and the sugar.
2. Open the cardamom pod, take out the seeds and crush them fine. Peel the ginger and grate fine. Add both to the hot orange juice.
3. Squeeze the gelatin (which should be marinated in water) and add to the juice.
4. Beat the marzipan into the mixture. Mix in the yogurt and allow to cool.
5. Beat the cream to soft peaks and fold in.
6. Fill the crème into four molds and place in the refrigerator until firm.

---

*Sheet gelatin is available at specialty food markets, or to convert to powdered gelatin, 3 sheets is equal to 4.5 grams or a little more than $^1/_2$ envelope of powdered gelatin.

Ginger Ice Cream

Serves 4.

4 egg yolks

$^2/_3$ cup sugar

$1^1/_4$ cups milk

$1^1/_4$ cups cream

2 tablespoons fresh ginger

2 tablespoons maple syrup

2 tablespoons honey

1 vanilla bean

4 fresh peppermint leaves

1. Beat the egg yolks with the sugar in a bowl until pale and thick.
2. Slowly heat the milk.
3. Add the cream to the egg yolks and then slowly mix in the warm milk.
4. Heat the mixture on low heat while stirring constantly. Do not let it boil.
5. Allow to cool and place in fridge.
6. Peel the ginger and grate fine. Add ginger, maple syrup, honey, and vanilla to the cooled custard.
7. Freeze the custard in an ice cream maker.
8. Divide the ice cream into four portions and decorate each with a peppermint leaf.

Index

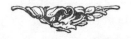